Praise ~~for~~ ~~Get~~ *he Stress*

"Risa Williams not only knows how to get stuff done, she makes it seem easy, simple, and fun to do! Williams's unique goal-mapping tools help us create what we want by being gentle and consistent with ourselves throughout the process and celebrating our accomplishments along the way. She encourages us to lean into a 'self-kindness mindset' vs. a 'toxic productivity' one, which is so important. Definitely a must-read book!"

—Eden Byrne, psychotherapist and EMDR practitioner

"This book is a must-read for anyone who struggles with burnout while working on goals. Risa Williams is an expert on a healthier and gentler approach to productivity, and *Get Stuff Done Without the Stress* has many practical tools and everyday mindset shifts for high achievers who also want to stay balanced across many areas of their lives."

—Sepideh Saremi, LCSW, founder of Run Walk Talk®

"This is a fantastic book that will teach you how to *Get Stuff Done Without the Stress*. Often people create a false dichotomy between either being productive or de-stressing. Risa Williams expertly teaches you how to work smarter, not harder. If you are feeling overwhelmed by both needing to get things done and the stress of everything, this book is for you!"

—Scott Waltman, president elect of the Academy of Cognitive & Behavioral Therapies and author of *The Stoicism Workbook*

"Powerful. Actionable. And entertaining! What more could you want from a book that helps you live your life purposes and reduce your stress? Highly recommended!"

—Eric Maisel, author of *Choose Your Life Purposes*

"Risa Williams has done it again! Williams expertly breaks down the science of getting things done into bitesize chunks, making it incredibly easy to immediately make significant changes in your life. In the current 'hustle climate,' it is refreshing to read an easy-to-follow blueprint for healthy productivity. As a psychologist, this book will be a go-to resource that I can share with clients struggling with burnout, procrastination, and the mindset of toxic productivity."

—Tamara Soles, PhD, psychologist

"Do you want to know a secret that will help you not only maximize your time but enjoy life more? Risa Williams shares *five* of them in her newest book, *Get Stuff Done Without the Stress*. Yes, she's done it again. This book is packed with tools, strategies, and insights on how to function well while getting things done effectively, providing a step-by-step pathway to freedom when you feel stuck, overwhelmed, or burnt out. There's help on every page! Living calmly enables us to be more productive and do better work. When you encourage yourself and enjoy the process, you get more done and feel better for it! One key strategy is practicing the feelings you want to feel before you experience them. The practical, tried-and-tested tools in this book make that possible. Want Future You to feel better than you do now and boost your productivity? Keep Calm and Read this Book!"

—Trevor Stockwell, author and leadership & personal development coach

"Risa is a talented clinician that has the unique ability to create tangible tools to help people get past their stuck points. The tools contained in her book, *Get Stuff Done Without the Stress*, are easily understandable and ready to be implemented. Risa makes the process of becoming a better version of yourself less daunting."

—Stevon Lewis, author and therapist

"As a tech founder constantly juggling high stakes and intense demands, Risa Williams has been a transformative resource in my life. Her insights and practical tools have not only helped me manage anxiety but also equipped me to break free from the grip of toxic productivity and resist the relentless hustle culture. Through her approach to mindfulness, boundary setting, and emotional resilience, I've become a more grounded and focused founder, which has enhanced my ability to lead with clarity and compassion. I especially appreciate how Risa integrates traditional cognitive behavioral therapy with therapeutic practices, creating a holistic toolkit that has empowered me to thrive and show up as a better leader."

—Ramona Ortega, Esq., CEO of WealthBuild.ai, leader of the THRIVE Campaign, public speaker, and fintech thought leader

"*Get Stuff Done Without the Stress* is a refreshingly compassionate approach to productivity that transforms how we think about managing our time and achieving our goals. Rather than pushing readers toward burnout through toxic hustle culture, Risa Williams offers a revolutionary framework built on self-kindness, combining her expertise as a psychotherapist with practical tools that help readers maintain balance while making meaningful progress. Through evidence-based techniques like the Task Intensity Meter, Small Steps Journal, and Morning Reset, Williams teaches us how to break down overwhelming goals into manageable pieces while actively reducing stress and expanding our capacity for calm. Her engaging writing style and relatable examples make complex concepts accessible, while her emphasis on treating ourselves with the same compassion we show others provides a sustainable foundation for long-term success. This isn't just another productivity book—it's a gentle but powerful guide to getting things done while protecting our well-being and finding genuine joy in our accomplishments."

—Dr. Christopher Cortman, author and psychologist

get
stuff
done

Without

THE
STRESS

A kinder approach to productivity

get stuff done

Without
THE
STRESS

5 **secrets** for making the best use of your time and achieving your **goals** for **greater happiness**

RISA WILLIAMS, LMFT

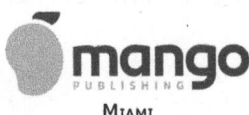

mango
PUBLISHING

MIAMI

For permission requests, please contact the publisher at:
Mango Publishing Group
5966 South Dixie Highway, Suite 300
Miami, FL 33143
info@mango.bz

For special orders, quantity sales, course adoptions and corporate sales, please email the publisher at sales@mango.bz. For trade and wholesale sales, please contact Ingram Publisher Services at customer.service@ingramcontent.com or +1.800.509.4887.

Getting Stuff Done Without the Stress: 5 Secrets for Making the Best Use of Your Time and Achieving Your Goals for Greater Happiness

Library of Congress Cataloging-in-Publication number: 2024947358
ISBN: (print) 978-1-68481-687-3, (ebook) 978-1-68481-688-0
BISAC category code: SEL024000, SELF-HELP / Self-Management / Stress Management

This book is for anyone who has ever felt completely overwhelmed, stressed out, and burnt out. I hope this book provides a little boost to help you discover what the next small step forward is for you.

Small steps add up, and you can figure things out, one small step at a time.

Table of Contents

Introduction

Where People Tend to Get Lost

Have you ever felt really overwhelmed and lost while trying to achieve your goals? Have you ever felt so stressed out by everyday tasks that you couldn't get started on any of them? Have you ever felt completely crushed by your to-do list to the point that you avoided looking at it for days on end?

Does even thinking about your weekly schedule right now fill you with an impending sense of doom and despair?

I know how you feel! I have often felt all these things myself, and I understand how easy it can be to get lost in burnout, overwhelm, frustration, and stress as you're working toward your goals. Every week, I help many different people from many different backgrounds and occupations, who are feeling extremely lost with their goals, find their way back on track again.

I'm a psychotherapist, psychology professor, time management coach, and book author who has written five self-help books exploring how to manage time in an easier way. In fact, I spend most of my time talking to people about time—how they want to spend their time, how they *don't* want to spend their time, and how they can create more time to do all the things they really want to do.

And we can do this together here in this book. To begin with, you can ask yourself these three time-related questions right now:

What things really matter to you that you would like to be spending more time on each day?

What things make you feel calm and happy, and how can you do more of these things each week?

What big goals are important to you that you would like to be taking regular steps toward each month?

And that's what we're about to figure out for you in chapters ahead. Using tools from cognitive behavioral therapy and behavioral science, mindfulness techniques, time management tools, and stress reduction strategies, let's start to figure out how to walk yourself over to your goals, one small step at a time.

However, getting to our goals doesn't really matter if we're seriously stressing ourselves out in the process. Everyday life is stressful enough to manage, why would we want to pile even more stress onto our plates?

There are already hundreds of unbalanced methods out there to become more manically productive, to frantically check off all the boxes, and to finish off your to-do list, all at the expense of your own mental, emotional, and physical well-being.

But honestly, who really wants all of that? Ideally, we want arriving at the finish line of our goals to make us feel *better*, not worse! And if we can't keep our brains and bodies balanced in pursuit of doing what we want to do, no matter what method or system we try, it just isn't going to be sustainable. We're going to be more prone to procrastinate, to stall out at the starting line, to burn out from exhaustion, to make ourselves sick in the process, or to give up on the process altogether, unless we're approaching our time in a calmer and healthier way.

Sometimes, our modern "hustle culture" can make us feel like we need to constantly push ourselves into a manic productivity mode in order to just keep up with what we think everyone else is doing. And along the way, it can be easy to lose track of our general well-being and what's really important to us in life. We can start to feel, as one client put it, like we're "running on a nonstop hamster wheel of stress."

As a therapist, I tend to see things from a different perspective. I look at goal setting from a "feelings" place instead of a "things" place.

In the grand scheme of things, we usually want to accomplish our goals because of the feelings we want to feel as a result of achieving them. In other words, it's not so much about getting to the *thing* as it is about getting to the *feeling* we think the *thing* will provide us with.

Think about this right now. Most of us are able to picture ourselves getting to our goals, but we can't often picture what we will feel after we get there. For example, perhaps you picture yourself completing a big goal like winning an award, buying a house, starting a business, taking a trip, or moving to a new city. You may see yourself in your "goal picture," but most likely, it isn't colored in with any emotions; it's just a picture of you doing a thing. You're holding a trophy, or a pair of keys, or standing somewhere, like on the top of a mountain you've just climbed.

It's just a picture without any feelings attached.

So, let's color in your "goal picture" right now with some really bright and vibrant feelings. What do you want to feel after you accomplish your goal?

Happy? Proud? Excited? Delighted? Joyful? Relieved? Grateful? Satisfied? Choose one of these feelings to focus on and try to feel it for a minute right now. Give yourself permission to fully feel it for a moment or two.

Notice how all you had to do was simply imagine yourself feeling this feeling for a second to actually experience a tiny burst of it. Now, walk yourself forward a few more steps in your mind and picture yourself a few weeks after you've completed your goal. What is Future You feeling, knowing that you have accomplished this goal? How does Future You feel going through everyday life?

As we practice the feelings we want to feel more intentionally throughout the course of this book, we will strengthen our ability to actually experience these feelings on a regular basis. These emotions are our goal, and we have to pave the pathway for our brains to get to these specific emotional destinations.

When we tell our brain where we want to go emotionally, our brain can help get us there.

The Nonstop Hamster Wheel

When I was a kid, you could say I was the textbook picture of the over-achieving stress case: winning competitions, scholarships, and awards; pushing myself way beyond the limits of what was manageable for me to do; and living in a constant state of anxiety as a result. Although I became very good at racking up a long list of achievements on paper, what I completely missed out on was feeling good about anything I was doing. In fact, the *more* I achieved, the *worse* I seemed to feel. And no matter how much I did, I never felt like I was doing *enough*.

This unhealthy pattern continued until my late thirties, when I somehow landed myself in the emergency room, knocked out from complete exhaustion, most likely as a result of my own extremely stressful approach to productivity. And it wasn't until I hit this serious low point, lying in a hospital bed, that I suddenly realized: *Something has to change. Somehow, I had the equation all wrong.*

Accomplishments really mean nothing if you wind up hurting your brain and body trying to achieve them. We need to *befriend* ourselves, not turn *against* ourselves in the pursuit of our goals.

What if this was actually our main life goal, to befriend ourselves? How many of us could say we have accomplished this particular goal? How differently would you approach things if you believed this to be true? What things would you decide to change in your life? What would you do differently from now on?

As I was having this intense moment of clarity in the hospital, my phone suddenly started to buzz with work requests from my supervisor, who knew I was in the emergency room yet was clearly not processing that I wouldn't be able to keep working despite being there.

Suddenly, I began to comprehend how absurd this whole situation truly was. I had overworked myself into the hospital, and now, work was trying to pull me out of the hospital just to put me back in there all over again! In that moment, I realized that if I wanted to get to a different outcome in the future, I had to change things, one step at a time, going forward.

Making a change was completely nonnegotiable.

And that's how I finally scared myself off the nonstop hamster wheel of stress.

In the years that followed, I slowly started to change the way I approached my own time. I decided that taking care of my brain and body was essential, because I couldn't do anything *without* them. I know this realization sounds obvious enough, but in reality, doing things differently becomes a daily practice once you fully accept this to be true.

Once you learn to be kinder to your brain and body on a regular basis, it changes many things you do, including what you decide to bring into and keep out of your life.

After all, you are in a long-term relationship with *yourself*. It's the most long-term committed relationship you will ever have with anyone. So, why not make it a friendly and loving one, going forward?

We Are Humans, Not Robots

When we're working on goals and projects in a healthy and balanced way, we can find our flow, which can lead us to feel a general sense of well-being. And that's what we're aiming for here in this book, to find that sense of life balance while working on things that are meaningful to us in some way.

However, when do things start to tip over into *toxic productivity* vs. *healthy productivity* as we're working on our goals? Throughout my own work and my work with many clients, I have discovered that there are many core beliefs around *toxic productivity* that are very common in our culture and can affect us and influence our behavior, whether we are conscious of them or not.

Here are a few examples. See which ones resonate with you:

Toxic Productivity Mindset

- You must work nonstop to get stuff done

- Producing output is the most important thing in life

- Resting is "lazy and non-productive" since it decreases output

- Progress is only measurable in output

- Success is only measured by how your output compares to other people's output

- You should stop at nothing until you accomplish big wins that will impress other people

- However, any "successes" should be downplayed so they do not ruffle the feathers of the people you were trying to impress (even though this directly contradicts the preceding rule)

- You must complete *everything* on your to-do list in order to feel "done" (never mind that you never stop adding new items to your to-do list)

- Showing yourself "tough love" by pushing through things when you're exhausted is the only way to increase your output

- When you're not working, you should feel guilty about not working, because it means you have not generated output

Reading this, doesn't it sound like it should be applied to some sort of factory robot versus a living human being? Unfortunately, many of us carry around these types of distorted beliefs throughout our lives, and they tend to affect how we feel about ourselves, each and every day!

In other words, these distorted core beliefs can make us feel bad a whole lot of the time. We feel bad when we do things and we feel bad when we rest. We don't give ourselves credit when we accomplish little things, but we don't give ourselves credit when we accomplish big things, either. When we take a vacation, we stress ourselves out about the work we're missing. And when we're working, we stress ourselves out about not taking more vacations. When we're at home, we can't connect with our loved ones because our to-do list is crowding out our thoughts. However, when we work on our to-do list, we tell ourselves we're dropping the ball on connecting with our loved ones.

Are you starting to see how deep all this goes?

As I started to slowly pull myself off of the nonstop hamster wheel of stress, I began to form a new concept of a *self-kindness mindset* as a way to approach our time and goals, one which looks at our whole lives through a new lens of general well-being.

Here are some of the key components of this *self-kindness mindset* when it comes to managing our time:

The Self-Kindness Mindset

- Our lives have many different areas that require balance in order for us to feel a sense of general well-being and happiness

- Rest when your brain and body need to rest

- Figuring out what you want to *feel* in the future helps you figure out what you want to *do*

- Downtime is not "lazy," it's a necessity; it helps our brains and bodies function

- Finding ways to connect to your calm is a daily practice that can help you manage your time more effectively

- Defining what your current core values are helps you find your motivation and focus

- Speaking to yourself in a kind and encouraging way helps you move forward

- There is no single way to accomplish a goal; you can create your own path and figure out your own small steps along the way

- Give yourself permission to feel "done" with things at the end of each day as a way to show yourself love, compassion, and kindness

- You can go at a pace that allows you to maintain your general well-being and balance

- You are on a lifelong learning journey, and you are always learning and growing

- Acknowledging what you've done is essential for your own growth, happiness, and self-esteem

- Showing yourself consistent kindness, care, and encouragement helps you get stuff done

Kindness *helps* you—if all you take away from this book is that being kinder to yourself will inevitably help you do everything you want to do, then that's a win right there!

As you continue through this book, it can be helpful to start to think about how you would like to redefine productivity for yourself. What is your new and healthier definition of productivity going to be from now on?

After practicing a **self-kindness mindset** for many years, the surprise twist was that I somehow became far more effective at getting stuff done as a result. Even though being productive wasn't my active main goal anymore, I was naturally accomplishing many more things in much shorter amounts of time, simply by showing myself more regular kindness, care, and compassion.

> *The more calm my life became, the more time seemed to stretch itself to suit my needs.*

However, you can't just teleport yourself there instantly from where you are now, if where you are now is feeling completely burnt out, beat up, overwhelmed, and exhausted. You have to figure it out at your own pace, one step at a time, and start to consistently increase your compassion and kindness toward yourself over a stretch of time.

Starting now, you can allow yourself to feel happy, to feel calm, to feel proud, and to feel good about yourself, no matter what you are doing or what steps you are taking. You can allow yourself to rest, to play, to have fun, and to choose to do things that really matter to you.

Your worth and value do not change because you do different things or move at different paces over time. You have intrinsic worth whether you are moving fast or slow, and whether you are resting, playing, or working. You are a human being, not a factory robot. And what an amazing thing it is to be alive! You can decide what is meaningful to you, and you can choose what you want to do with your time here.

Sometimes, we just forget we have a choice!

Throughout this book, it is my hope that you will learn to adopt a **self-kindness mindset** when it comes to your time and your goals. Once you do, your relationship with time will also start to shift in a more positive direction as well. It's just what starts to happen naturally, even if all you're doing is showing yourself more kindness and compassion each day.

How Burnout Begins

While the levels of burnout and exhaustion I experienced don't always land people in the emergency room, they are unfortunately not all that uncommon for most people these days.

Brain Boost:

According to the latest Gallup news survey, 49 percent of Americans are feeling chronically high levels of stress, which marks a sixteen-point increase over the last twenty years. Women are feeling higher "everyday" stress levels than ever, with 53 percent of American women reporting higher daily stress levels than men. And in terms of burnout, 70 percent of workers polled across seven countries reported feeling "burnt out" on a regular basis, with extremely "low levels of emotional well-being," in a recent study done by Asana.

I would even venture to say that feeling burnt out is more the norm than not these days, and that's even more of a reason to learn to utilize the tools in this book right now to find your way back into balance again.

Over the years, I've found that it's altogether too common for people to accomplish really big things yet feel nothing emotionally as a result. I have witnessed so many people complete truly impressive goals, only to deny themselves any feelings of pride, happiness, or relief afterwards. Forget doing that victory dance at the touchdown line, they often don't even acknowledge *anything* that they have achieved, even if it's something that's taken them years to complete!

Instead, after we accomplish a goal, there is often a persistent feeling of *"that's done, now what?"* This feeling tends to prod us toward the next goal-carrot-on-a-stick, which we then just keep moving further and further down the line. We may tell ourselves, *"When I get to this next thing, then I will* really *feel happy,"* only when we get to that thing, we just plug in the next thing, and the thing after that, and we never really allow ourselves to feel happy or proud about anything we've just completed or any of the steps along the way.

> *Ask yourself: When was the last time I felt really happy*
> *or proud of something I did?*

Remember those goals we were talking about—starting businesses, buying houses, going on trips, and so on? When people accomplish these types of big goals, they finally get to step inside of that "goal picture" they previously imagined inside their heads. However, often the feelings don't match the picture at all; people often feel far more exhausted and worn-out as a result of pushing for so long to get to their goal. Also, the rest of their life may have really been thrown off-balance as a result of all that pushing, so it can feel chaotic and stressful, rather than joyful and exciting.

In other words, their "goal picture" doesn't always feel all that happy to them in reality, when they finally get to step inside of it!

Ideally, we want the feelings to match the goal we just completed. We want to feel happy and proud; we want to look back and think, *"Look at all those steps I just took to get here. Look how far I have come from where I started! That's amazing!"*

In order for this to happen, we have to pave the emotional pathway for our brains to get there, each tiny step of the way. We have to train our brains to feel proud of what we're doing as we're doing it, when we're in the middle of it, and after we've completed it altogether.

Think of this type of self-encouragement as a muscle: You have to build it with exercise and training until one day that muscle becomes very, very strong. And once that muscle is strong, nothing can stop you from cheering yourself on. You'll do it automatically. You'll cheer yourself on when you wash the dishes. You'll give yourself a pat on the back when you send off an email. You'll encourage yourself the whole way through, for little things and big things, easy things and hard things. And then, your confidence in your ability to do more amazing things will naturally start to grow.

When we don't acknowledge what we have completed, this communicates to our brain that there is absolutely no emotional reward for finishing all the challenging things we've just walked ourselves through. After this lack of acknowledgment, is it any wonder that the next time you're at the starting line of another new and intimidating goal, your brain doesn't want to sign up for taking the first step forward?

"Where's the emotional reward?" it asks; "How will we feel any better after doing all these difficult and uncomfortable things we're about to do? In fact, why not just stay right here in one place instead?"

This is how we sometimes wind up getting stuck in procrastination or find ourselves drifting off from projects we really want to do. We lose our motivation and energy to take on yet another challenge because our brain has predicted that the emotional outcome will not be beneficial for us to experience.

So, as we move forward in this book, let's discover a kinder, gentler, more encouraging way to get stuff done, and let's tailor it just for you. After all, everyone's brain is different. We need to take the time with the tools in this book to try things out, experiment, and tinker with ideas until we find the right combination that works for your own particular brain.

We can be kind toward ourselves in this process, and in the long run, we'll develop a practical system that you can use consistently for many years after you're done with this book.

Going forward, let's aim for getting stuff done in a healthier and happier way from now on.

How This Book Works

In my experience of working with many different people over the years, I've found that there are *five main factors* that can help us feel more in control of our time, goals and happiness. I've designed the book to focus on these five factors, providing practical, simple, and easy tools that you can use in everyday situations right now.

While reading through the chapters ahead, you inevitably may bump into harsh self-talk you didn't know was occurring, or gain greater insight about the everyday stress you're under, or discover that there are deeper layers to why you are feeling stuck with things. It's always recommended that you seek out help from a professional, a doctor or a therapist, to help you process any intense emotions, patterns, or stuck points you might be experiencing right now.

This book is intended as a supplemental tool, and it is not a replacement for therapy or medical advice. It is simply meant to provide new and creative ideas that can hopefully help you start to shift your approach to managing your time and goals in a gentler way. When used in conjunction with regular therapy or coaching, these tools can often turbo-boost your motivation and momentum forward.

After completing each chapter, you will unlock a new key that will help you understand the next chapter going forward. In this way, each chapter's tools build upon each other, so it makes the most sense to read the book in the order it was written. Take it one technique at a time, one section at a time, one day at a time. There's no need to rush through everything in a big hurry.

In fact, that "go-go-go rush-rush-rush" mentality is one we're actively trying to move away from in this book. We can slow down the pace a little as we read these pages so that we can let it all in. This way, by the time you get to the end of the book, I'm hoping you will have collected a few key insights that will have you looking at your time and yourself through a much kinder lens.

Here are the five stages of this book:

1. **Mapping Out Goals:** In this chapter, we start with a creative warm-up exercise that gets you to map out your goals on paper and figure out what the next easy step forward is for you. Goals can sometimes feel like amorphous blobs floating around in our heads, undefined by actionable steps or realistic time frames, and this technique will help make them more tangible to you. It's going to give you that much-needed motivational boost forward into the next chapters of the book and onto the path toward your goals.

2. **Creating Calm:** This chapter teaches us how to find our calm and balance while we're navigating our goal path. In order to get stuff done *without* the stress, we really need to assess how much stress we're currently under right now and what types of tasks are stressing us out the most. As we learn to expand our capacity for calm, we also learn to stretch out our perception and experience of time. In other words, we can create more time for ourselves to get stuff done by finding ways to consistently connect with our calm each day.

3. **Designing Time:** Now that we've created space for calmer feelings, how can we create actual space in our schedule each week to get stuff done? Creating space is more than just leaving a few hours free in your calendar

to methodically plug in tasks and projects; it's an entire mindset shift that will get you looking at your week ahead from this perspective: "What is really important to me this week, and how can I protect it?" It's how we draw lines around our time. How do we create space to focus, to work on projects, to rest, to play, to reset, to experiment, to have fun? What are the things that are meaningful to us that we are going to make space for this week in our calendar?

4. **Showing Yourself Proof:** We've now created space *and* time to get stuff done, now comes the most important part. How do we show our brains proof that we're making progress on our goals? It's one thing to robotically check off your to-do list, it's another thing to feel really good about all the things you're checking off. We need to prove to your brain that you're making progress each week so that you can *allow* yourself to feel good about all the tiny steps you're taking along the way. This chapter will teach you how to befriend yourself during all phases of progress.

5. **Embracing Being "Done":** Here's the real gist of why you wanted to read this book. You want to feel happy after you've completed things. You want to feel done! Really and truly happy and done. In this chapter, we'll walk over to that "happy and done" feeling, and we'll look at how you can allow yourself to savor it a little more deliberately.

Before you picked up this book, you had probably already experimented with many different time management systems that worked for a little while and then didn't, and you've also probably tried many techniques that never worked for you at all. While the tools in this book may seem very simple at first, I've witnessed hundreds of different people effectively applying them in hundreds of different ways. These tools are adaptable and flexible to suit your ever-changing schedule, lifestyle, and needs. And flexibility really is the key to getting into a happier flow with your time on a regular basis.

It's never too late, or even too early, to start figuring out ways to make friends with time.

After all, we only have so much time on this planet, how do we want to be spending it?

Let's find out!

Chapter One

Map Out Your Goals: Three Is the Magic Number

You Need a Map

You know how in adventure movies, there will typically be a moment where the protagonist becomes really lost and confused about what to do next? Our hero doesn't quite know how to proceed, so they enlist the help of someone who sweeps everything off the table in front of them, plops down a map, and starts drawing stuff out with a marker, saying matter-of-factly, "So, here's what we're going to do next..." while inspiring music starts to play? And then, you know it's going to be okay somehow, that the hero will be off on the adventure soon in the upbeat montage that will inevitably follow?

Growing up, I always admired that "table sweeper" character, whenever I watched these types of adventure movies. I wanted to meet this person in real life, someone armed with markers to start mapping things out with me. There were so many times during my adult years where I wished a "table sweeper" would magically appear and boldly announce, "Now, here's what we're going to do next..." as I toiled away at a demoralizing job or fumbled my way through projects I didn't know how to complete. Because I really could have used their help when faced with the many roadblocks and stuck points that popped up throughout everyday life.

But this didn't happen to me in reality. Although I had some wonderful mentors sprinkled into life here and there, it was much more of a messy, confusing, nebulous, and stressful process for me to navigate my way toward my goals, big or small. I often felt lost more often than I felt clear and focused about what I was doing or where I was going next. Perhaps you can relate to this?

I am guessing most of us didn't have "table sweepers" magically show up as we made our way through adulthood, getting more and more lost in our own emotional fogs as we worked toward our goals.

That's why here in this book, I'm going to teach you how to be *your own* table sweeping mentor. I'm going to teach you how to map things out on paper so you can walk yourself over to your goals, one small step at a time.

Mapping It Out

Your Goals Map: Using my **Goal-Mapping System**, we're going to map out our goals from a higher level perspective, making sure we're maintaining our emotional, mental, and physical balance across all of them as we're planning them out. Then, we can begin to break those big goals into tiny easy steps until we find the first steps forward, so we can start to feel more motivated to take on the journey ahead.

End of the Month Review: At the end of the month, we'll look back on what we've done, where we've gotten off-balance with things, and what adjustments we want to make going forward. Sometimes, we might want to swap out goals for other ones as we get more clarity on how we want to direct our energy. At other times, we may get more information that helps fine-tune our path. All of this requires monthly reflection that can wind up being something you actually might start to look forward to doing, because you will learn that it keeps you from tipping yourself over into stress more regularly.

Roadblocks and Rest Stops: Once we develop an understanding of which goal columns we're working on, we can learn to pace ourselves with more kindness along the way. When one goal column naturally hits a bump in the road or a stopping point, we can figure out how to balance ourselves out by taking breaks or by working on another column's small steps forward.

Besides clarifying our intentions going forward, doing this also helps to keep things feeling fun and inspiring for us to do.

Our brains need a mix of fun, flexibility, and focus to stay motivated on the path toward our goals.

When we become overly strict and rigid in our goal setting, we can short-circuit the fun right out of the entire process. This can include making our deadlines too intense and too short, putting excessive pressure on ourselves to make huge instant leaps forward, expecting ourselves to do each step "perfectly" and "flawlessly," and not giving ourselves enough downtime and relaxation along the way.

We're trying to avoid becoming harsh goal enforcers or taskmasters by using a system that allows us to visually acknowledge the different areas we're working on each month in a way that will help us keep things in balance.

By keeping our balance when working on goals,
we can connect with the fun of doing them.

Learning these **Goal-Mapping** tools can help you become the table sweeping mentor that you've always wished would appear in your own life. You'll learn where you tend to get stuck along the way and practice creative strategies for getting motivated again. You'll start to learn how to pull back and see your progress from a higher level perspective, as though you are watching yourself traveling down a path toward things you want to achieve.

Getting this new *map view* will help you really start to appreciate everything you've already done, everything you're doing right now, and everything you're about to do next.

You're going to become a steady and supportive witness to your very own goals journey from now on, and you'll start to see how exciting this can be.

So, are you ready? Let's sweep off that table (as dramatically as you want to), roll out some paper, grab some markers, and get started. Cue up that inspiring music, and let's go!

Make the Intangible Tangible

Goals can sometimes feel like amorphous clouds floating above our heads that follow us around, telling us we need to take immediate action now, when we don't really know what that action *is*. And then, we tend to beat ourselves up unfairly because we can't get started, which seems like a really harsh thing to do;

after all, how can we take that first step forward if we've never defined what that step actually is?

This was the case for one of the very first clients who came to work with me on goal setting. He said he had been "burning out" and beating himself up trying to launch his own creative business, and he looked really exhausted. He was trying to leave a job in advertising to launch a business doing graphic design, but even the mere idea of his new goal was making him feel overwhelmed and stuck, and he was "losing lots of sleep over it."

He hadn't taken the first step forward because he didn't know what that was, and he was full of "self-doubt" and "frustration" over not being able to figure it all out.

"I should have started my business years ago," he said, "I don't know why I haven't done it already."

He said he knew "in his heart" that it was now time to start moving toward his goals or else, "I'm going to wake up in ten years and wonder why I am still working at a job I can't stand, one that's taking up all the time I want to be using for other things that are much more important to me. I'm going to look back and wonder, 'Why didn't I just start when I had the chance?' "

After listing out everything he wanted to do in the future, he sighed and said, "I just wish there was a map to help me get to where I want to go and tell me what the next step ahead is that I'm supposed to take. But as a grown-up, there really is no map, is there?"

I paused for a few seconds, considered what he had just said, and then told him, "Well, I guess you'll have to make one, then."

While I didn't sweep a table off dramatically, I did pull out a blank piece of paper and hand it to him. As a therapist, I learned early on to always have a blank pad of paper on hand for clients to write things out on, because I discovered that it generally helps people organize their ideas, while also bringing their stress down a little.

I offered him my pen, but instead, he said, "Hang on a second."

He then opened up his backpack and produced a neat set of markers all bundled up together, and held them up proudly for me to see, which made me laugh.

"You carry around markers with you?" I asked.

"Yes, and..." then he produced a ruler out of the same backpack, which made me laugh some more.

"And a ruler, too?"

"For moments like this, I guess," he laughed; "I told you I was an artist, right?"

After a minute of neatly arranging his art supplies on the coffee table, he looked up excitedly and asked, "So, what's next?"

"Let's just start mapping things out on paper and see where it goes," I replied, and I watched as we started to fill up the page.

From that day forward, I've been mapping things out with clients. And as a result, I've been fortunate enough to witness many different people moving forward with their goals, including that particular artist, who wound up launching a very successful business which he still runs to this day.

After many years of using it, I named this tool **Goal-Mapping**. It's become the easiest way for clients to keep track of what they're working on each month and to find those first steps forward while also maintaining their general well-being.

So, how do we go about finding our balance while working on our goals and how do we figure out what the first step forward is?

Three Is the Magic Number

A lot of people tend to approach goal setting in *extremes*. They either get overly fixated on accomplishing a gigantic mono-goal that consumes all of their energy, time, and attention (often to the detriment of other areas in their life that quickly descend into chaos), or they want to work on so many dozens of scattered goals across so many scattered categories that they completely overwhelm themselves into not doing *any* of them. I call this the **everything, everywhere, all at once** problem. Do you ever catch yourself doing something like this?

For instance, clients will often say things like, "Well, I have to get in shape, get a new career, find a new partner, finish that creative project, and move to a new place..." and then they will add this extra little piece of stress: "...*in the next month.*"

Whether they're trying to tackle dozens of scattered goals all at once or become overly focused on a gigantic mono-goal, there's often far too much urgency to achieve their goals instantly, which winds up shutting people down completely, rather than moving them forward at all.

To visualize these two types of "extreme goal setting" that people tend to do with their goals, you can look at it like this:

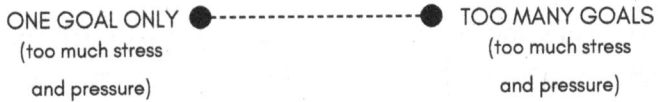

ONE GOAL ONLY ●--------------------● TOO MANY GOALS
(too much stress   (too much stress
and pressure)   and pressure)

What's the secret to keeping your balance with goals? I've found through working with many different people that *three is the magic number* for working on manageable and reasonable goals each month. Notice that the key words are *manageable* and *reasonable*, which means we are breaking our goals down into smaller steps so we can pace ourselves in a calmer and more balanced way.

Instead of putting so much unnecessary stress and pressure on ourselves to accomplish our goals "instantly," we're going to try to find a steady and consistent pace that works for us to maintain our general life balance instead. We're taking things in small steps and watching how all of these small steps walk us over to really big things over time.

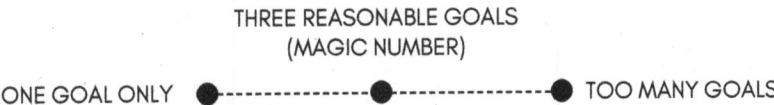

THREE REASONABLE GOALS
(MAGIC NUMBER)

ONE GOAL ONLY ●--------------●--------------● TOO MANY GOALS

You can do really big things if you break those big things down into tiny steps and take those tiny steps consistently, at a pace that feels manageable to you.

Map It Out

To begin using this **Goal-Mapping** tool, we are going to focus on *three areas of your life* where you are going to set goals. You're going to be working on these goals for the next few months, and we're going to break each of your three goals down into weekly steps you can take moving forward.

On a piece of paper, draw *three vertical columns*. Each column represents a goal that you would like to work on for the next few months.

In a minute, you will label the first two columns, but for now, move over to the third column, which we are going to label *"Self-Care"* at the top.

It should look like this:

THREE TRACK: GOALS

			SELF-CARE

As we will learn later in Chapter Two, which is titled *"Self-Care is Nonnegotiable,"* regulating our stress is essentially how we're going to more effectively manage our time from now on. This is why Column Three is already given the heading of "Self-Care."

The purpose of this *self-care track* is to *actively bring our stress down* in a regular and consistent way. In other words, these are activities in this column we're choosing to do regularly that will help us find our calm on a consistent basis.

Which activities work best for you to bring down your daily stress? To figure this out, you can ask yourself a few simple questions.

Ask yourself:
What activities tend to bring my stress down?
What activities help me connect with calm feelings?
What activities help me stay mentally, emotionally, and physically balanced each week?
What activities make me feel happy?

Across the last decade, many neuroscience studies[11] have shown that these types of activities tend to help people regulate their daily stress:

- Meditating

- Walking

- Exercising

- Practicing mindfulness

- Breathing techniques

- Being around "green spaces" (such as nature, trees, plants, forests, parks, hills)

---

1   [1] (Akimbekov NS, 2021), (Balban, MY, *et al*, 2023), (Can YS, *et al*, 2020), (Harvard University, 2021), (Kok, BE, *et al*, 2013), (White, MP, *et al*, 2021), (University of West England, 2018).

- Being around "blue spaces" (these include oceans, lakes, marinas, rivers, and pools of water)

- Listening to calming and soothing sounds and/or music

- Finding relaxing activities that engage your focus (such as drawing, journaling, and crafts)

- Sensory activities that engage our senses in a calming way

- Somatic relaxation techniques (stretches, breathwork, humming, movement)

- Healthy habits, including healthy eating, getting enough sleep, and regular exercise

- Grounding techniques that connect our brains to our bodies

We'll explore more of these stress-reducing techniques in Chapter Two, but for now, take some time to write down a few easy *self-care activities* that might work for you to do each week. Give your brain some flexible self-care options that are things you can do on your own, without too much planning or effort. For instance, if I put "going for a walk" as my top choice, what will I do when it rains or when I have a cold? In this case, I could add things like "listen to relaxing music" or "meditate" or "write in my journal," as this gives me a few options to pick from when my stress starts to rise.

A gentle reminder: This self-care goal column is about actively bringing our stress down. Therefore, make sure the things you're writing in this column feel manageable, calm, healthy, and easy for you to do.

What stress-reducing options will you put in your self-care column? Write them down under Column Three.

Naming Your Other Columns

Now let's figure out what we want to call Columns One and Two.

> *Ask yourself: What two goals do I want to work on for the next few months?*

You can select whatever two categories you would like to focus on right now, during this next period of time. Many clients tend to pick things like "Work Goals" and "Creative Projects" as their two columns, while other clients will choose things like: "House Projects," "Hobbies," "Organization Projects," "Relationships," "Family," or "Travel" for their columns instead. Other clients have created columns like "Socializing" to focus on proactively reaching out to more friends, "Grown-Up Stuff" for handling appointments, maintenance tasks, and household projects, or "Education" for learning new skills online. It's entirely up to you! You can call your two columns whatever you like.

Here is an example of what one client chose for her three columns:

THREE TRACK: GOALS

WORK	CREATIVE	SELF-CARE

What will you call your Column One and Column Two?

Time Frames for Your Three Columns

Now that we've named your three columns, we can start to figure out what a *reasonable and manageable* time frame is for you to do your goals in.

> *Ask yourself: What time frame feels reasonable for me to complete these goals in?*

Here's an example of how figuring out reasonable time frames for goals can look very different for three different people who all have the very same goal of writing a novel.

Client One has a goal of finishing her novel because she has sold her book to a publisher and the complete first draft is due in six months. In this case, her time frame is easy to lock down because the deadline has already been pre-established for her. She feels this deadline is reasonable for her because she has written a few other books before, and because she has finished large portions of the current one already. Her goal column would look like this:

Client One's Column

Column One: Write novel.
Six Month Goal: Turn in first draft of novel to publisher.

Now, let's take another person with the very same goal. Client Two is writing a novel in his spare time while also working a very busy full-time job. He has no established deadline for finishing his book other than what he would like to set for himself. He's never written a novel before, but he has completed many short stories. When Client Two is asked, "What is a reasonable time frame for this goal?" he thinks it will take him one year to complete a rough draft of his book if he writes for a few nights each week. His column would look like this:

Client Two's Column

Column One: Write novel.
One Year Goal: Finish rough draft of novel.

And now, let's take another person with the same goal. Client Three is trying to graduate with a university degree and write a novel at the same time. She also has a part-time job, so she is struggling to find time to write. She has never written a novel before and doesn't know how long it will take her to get it done. When asked what a "reasonable" time frame is for her goal, she decides that she has too much on her plate to finish the book any time soon, but in the next three months, she thinks she wants to complete an outline just to "get her ideas out on paper."

Client Three's Column

Column One: Write novel.
Three Month Goal: Write a simple outline.

You can see that for three different people who have a very similar goal, their goal steps and reasonable goal time frames all look very different from each other. You have to figure out what goal time frame is reasonable for *you*, considering all the other responsibilities and commitments you have going on during this period of time.

Whenever possible, try to give yourself *more than enough* time to accomplish your goals, especially for bigger goals. When we give yourself a longer stretch of time to complete things, it tends to lower our stress, rather than spiking it.

How We Break It Down

Now that we've established our goal time frame, we can break down the goal steps on paper. Let's take Client Three's goals and write them out in a **Goals Map**.

For example, with this client, I might ask her, "In three months' time, what do you want to have completed across all three of your columns?" She would answer, "I want to graduate, write my outline for my novel, and make sure that I am meditating, journaling, or going for walks each week more consistently to keep my stress down."

So, her map would start out looking like this:

THREE COLUMNS: GOALS

SCHOOL	CREATIVE	SELF-CARE
3 Months:	3 Months:	3 Months:
Graduate School	Write Outline	Meditating, journaling or walking three times per week

Funnel It Down

Once we have our *three goal columns* on an established time frame (three months, in this client's case), we can now begin the process of *funneling down* the columns. We want to move *from the future end date to the present* as we break our goals down into smaller steps across chunks of time.

Imagine a *goal funnel*. You put in a bigger goal at the top, and then, it goes down through the funnel, and eventually, a *small weekly goal step* comes out at the bottom. You can visualize it like this:

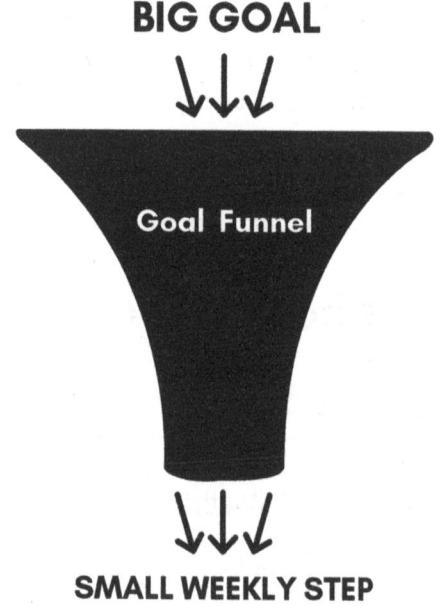

BIG GOAL

Goal Funnel

SMALL WEEKLY STEP

What does this look like on paper? Here is an example from this client:

SCHOOL	CREATIVE	SELF-CARE
3 Months:	3 Months:	3 Months:
Graduate School	Write Outline	Meditating, journaling or walking three times per week
One Month:	One Month:	One Month:
Finish writing final paper and take exams	Write half the outline	Meditating, journaling or walking one time per week
This Week:	This Week:	This Week:
Finish reading chapter of textbook	Journal about ideas on paper	Go for a walk on Friday

We're breaking things down on paper, going backward from the *end point of the goal* to the *present moment* in defined chunks of time. This is how we start to make the intangible more tangible to our brains, and it's also how we can start to visualize pacing ourselves in a manageable and reasonable way. Working backward helps us connect the dots and visually process the journey ahead of us.

Essentially, you're getting really honest with yourself by writing these things down. It's like telling yourself, *"Okay, you really want to do this thing? Here's what we're going to do next."* Your brain can now get a little more excited and a little less anxious about starting this new adventure with you.

If you're having trouble establishing a time frame for your columns, you can start with a time frame of three months just to practice using the tool, as that is usually an amount of time people can easily break down on paper. Even if your goal won't be completely finished in three months' time, most people can picture how much they might be able to reasonably do across their three columns during that amount of time.

Remember: *We're trying to avoid being harsh taskmasters while setting these goals, so make what you need to do in three months' time feel manageable to your own brain.*

Answer these questions:

- What do you want to have completed on each of your columns in three months' time? Write it down underneath all your columns under the heading: **Three Months**.

- Then, walk yourself backward to one month from now. Ask yourself: Where do you want to be with these goals in your columns in one month's time? Write it down under the heading: **One Month**.

- And now, walk yourself backward to this week. What needs to happen this week as your very first step forward for each of these columns? Write it down and define this step for yourself with the heading: **This Month**.

Working on Bigger Goals

For clients who are working with me on bigger goals, we typically start with a *one-year time frame* for their columns. Then each week, we check in on what tiny steps they have taken across all of their goal columns and adjust things on a regular basis. This process can help people understand that for bigger goals, they're going to need to give themselves a much longer stretch of time for completion so that they can pace themselves in a more balanced way. For people working on bigger goals with a *one-year time frame*, they would break it down on paper like this:

One year →Six months →Three months → One month → This week

If your goal has a shorter time frame, such as one month, you would break it down like this:

One month → Mid-month → This week

No matter what your established time frame is, you will always write out a *weekly goal step* at the bottom of each column. In this client's case, she decided on taking a walk, journaling about her outline, and finishing reading a chapter of her textbook as her first *weekly goal steps*.

These weekly goal steps should feel very small and easy for you to do. After all, the easier they sound, the more likely you will be to do them!

The First Step Forward

Our brains are like computers, and in order to program our brains to move forward with any of our goal columns, we need to break things down into *small actionable commands* for our brains to follow, starting with that very first one.

When we don't clearly define what that very first step is for ourselves, our brains may get stuck in the "spinning wheel" stage for a really long time; this is a state where we avoid and resist moving forward into the unfamiliar and unknown. It can therefore be helpful to make that first step sound as easy as possible to do so that our brains will get on board with taking it.

You can remember it like this:

> *The first step forward is the hardest part, so make it super easy for your brain to start.*

In fact, make that first step forward sound so very easy that it's difficult *not* to take it. Make it sound *ridiculously* easy, in fact!

Finding the First Step

Here are some examples of how clients discovered the easiest first step forward with their goals:

Goal: Painting a portrait
First Step: Put paintbrushes out on the table so I see them and remember to use them.

Goal: Finish work report
First Step: Open up the document and type one sentence of the report.

Goal: Go hiking on Tuesday
First Step: Tuesday morning, put hiking shoes by the door.

Goal: Sew my own jacket
First Step: Take the sewing machine out of the garage and move it to the living room.

Goal: Do yoga routine after work
First Step: Roll out the yoga mat onto the floor before leaving for work.

Goal: Learn new music software
First Step: Open up the music software and click on a few buttons.

To begin any goal:

- Figure out your reasonable and manageable time frame

- Break the goal down into manageable steps, starting from the end to the beginning in steps

- Define what the very easiest first step forward is

- When in doubt, write it out

Make the intangible more tangible by writing things out on paper to help yourself visually process the journey you're about to take. Show your brain the map, and your brain can rev up the engine to drive you there.

The Magic Post-it

Since the first steps forward are often the hardest ones for people to take, let's find a simple system to get your brain to remember to take those first steps this week.

Looking at your goals map, *circle the first weekly steps* at the bottom of the columns. Here's a sample of how that looks from the client in the example above:

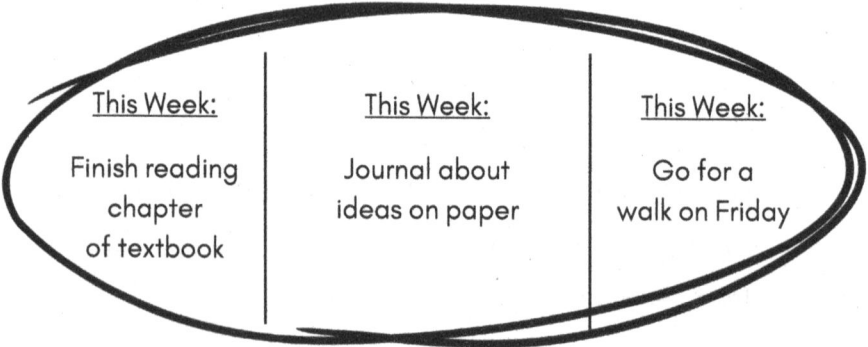

These are our *three main goal steps* for this week. We have now given ourselves actionable weekly steps that feel easy and manageable for us to do.

Now, we can transfer these weekly steps onto something I call **"The Magic Post-it."** This tool was originally called **"The Weekly Post-it,"** but a client wanted to rename it **"The Magic Post-it"** because he claimed, "It works like magic! I don't know how, but I always get things done when I write them on the Post-it each week."

Using a sticky note in a bright color, write out your *three weekly steps* in a simplified bullet list. It has to be a Post-it rather than a piece of paper. This is because we want to keep this particular list very short and simple going forward, so we are intentionally limiting the space where we're writing things out. A sticky note is usually the best way to do this since other, bigger pieces of paper will very quickly start to make things jumbled up. Also, there's a neurological reason that supports writing it out on paper as opposed to typing it out on a computer: Making notes by hand helps our brains retain the information more effectively.

Brain Boost:

In a recent study done at the Norwegian University of Technology, researchers tested the memories of student participants who could either write words down or type them to memorize them. They found that writing by hand helped participants remember the words better. Researchers stated: "For all the participants, writing by hand led to an increase in connectivity between central parts of the brain and the parietal lobe in the outer part of the brain, with the same not being true for typing." Dr. Audrey van der Meer concluded, "Handwriting uses more senses, and the body is more involved. That means more of the brain is active and there needs to be more communication in these active parts (of the brain)" (Ly, Chen, 2024).

So, let's help our brains out a little more by writing out a **Magic Post-it** for the week and prioritizing what needs to happen next in a way that we can remember it. Here's an example of how to do it from the goal steps of the client mentioned earlier:

Weekly Post-It

- Finish reading chapter

- Journal about ideas for outline

- Friday: Go for a walk

Now that you've written it out, place your Post-it in a place where you will actually see it every day. For years, I've been putting my **Magic Post-it** on my desk lamp right beside my computer. I have to look at it every time I sit down at my desk, which is usually multiple times per day, and I find that this visual repetition helps program my brain to remember what I need to focus on that particular week.

The client who renamed this tool **"The Magic Post-it"** explains, "After I write the three things down and put it on my desk, my brain then automatically knows to do them. No matter how busy I become, I somehow remember to do my weekly steps. Usually, I find that by Friday, I've done all the things on my Post-it, and if I haven't, it's easy for me to know what I need to catch up with on Monday. But most of the time, I've finished them all without thinking about it too much. It works like magic for me!"

For your **weekly Post-it** to work like "magic" for you, here are some simple rules to follow:

The Magic Post-it Rules:

- Each week, write your *three weekly goal steps* on your Post-it.

- As you accomplish each weekly step, cross it off and tell yourself, "I did it!"

- When you have finished everything on your Post-it, throw it away in the trash triumphantly!

Anything you don't finish by Friday gets carried over to next Monday's Post-it. In this way, you will quickly learn to catch up with the tasks you didn't do last week, since you can't add that many more tasks until you first clear off the ones on your current Post-it. The more you use this tool, the more you'll want to finish the items on your **Magic Post-it**, because it feels *really good* to throw that finished note away. So, slam-dunk it right into the trash when you're done. You did it! Now you can let yourself feel done for the week.

The Brain Dump List

So, what do you do about all those other "general miscellaneous life things" you need to do other than your *three weekly goals*? Most of us have many more than three things to do each week, so where do we put all of these other things we need to remember? Let's learn to separate out our lists, keeping our **"Magic Post-it"** as short as possible while allowing ourselves to keep a separate, slightly longer list in a notebook, which will be called "**The Brain Dump List**."

Separating out our **brain dump list** from our "**Magic Post-it**" will keep us from bumping into the main problems that people face due to keeping one master to-do list:

- Their to-do list is overwhelmingly long.

- Their to-do list is a jumbled mess of big things, small things, random things, important things, nonimportant things, and urgent things that must happen immediately.

When your brain has to read through a long, jumbled up to-do list like this, it won't know which task to prioritize next, it won't know how to sort any of it visually, and it won't know what's important to do this week; and as a result, it will start to feel really overwhelmed, really fast.

A rule of thumb: If you can see it in a simple way, you will probably do it. Ideally, we should be able to visually "scoop up" the bullet points on our Magic Post-it in one quick glance. With clear visual cues, we will be more likely to retain the information and act upon it.

Separating out visually what needs to happen *now* vs. what needs to happen *at some point in the future* helps your brain understand where to direct its focus next.

In other words, *curate* the information you're showing your own busy brain a little more intentionally each week.

Whittle It Away

Ideally, we don't want our **brain dump list** to get much longer than a page, or else we'll find ourselves back where we started, with an overwhelmingly long to-do list that just keeps stressing us out. So, how do we keep it down to one single page? By tackling one item off our **brain dump list** each week and by not allowing ourselves to add *any new items* until we have taken one off the list first.

Each week, pick one or two items off your **brain dump list** to add to the bottom of your weekly Post-it to complete. For example, in this client's case, she chose "paying her car registration fee" to put on her weekly Post-it, which looked like this:

<u>Weekly Post-It</u>

- Finish reading chapter

- Journal about ideas
  for outline

- Friday: Go for a walk

- Send in car registration fee
  by Wednesday

If you find you are falling really behind on your **brain dump list** items at the end of the month, you can swap out one of your main columns on your goals map to catch up on these items, as another client did with his "Grown-Up Stuff" column. By making his miscellaneous items a priority for the month, he was able to catch up on completing a few big list items that had been nagging at him for a long time, which gave him a huge sense of relief.

However, most of the time, if you're whittling away at your **brain dump list** at a slow and steady pace by doing a few small items per week, you'll be able to keep your list in check without too much effort.

When You Have a Really Busy Week

When things get really busy across multiple areas of your life, you may need to do a **daily Post-it** for a while instead of a weekly one. This requires scheduling a little time each morning to write out your daily Post-it ahead of time before you start on your day's tasks. The same rule applies: Try to focus on which *three things need to happen each day* and limit your Post-it to only these things.

Going forward, from now on, don't try to keep it all in your head all the time. Write it out on paper, and help your brain out a little more. You can remember it like this:

Do something today that helps Future You out
in some way.

Don't dump all the hard stuff on Future You to have to figure out later. Future You won't be able to magically solve all the problems you're pushing off into the future and definitely won't have any more motivation than Today You has right now. If anything, Future

You will have *less* motivation than you do now, since the more we avoid things, the more stressful they tend to become in the future.

So, put it down on paper now and make it easy for yourself *today*, and then Future You can help you out by doing the next tasks ahead in the future.

Be kind to Today You *and* Future You.

Just be kind to yourself *relentlessly*, from now on.

The Monthly Review

At the end of each month, you can review your goal map, swap out columns for new ones, choose your next small steps forward, and make any adjustments as needed. This is necessary to do so that you can reevaluate where you want to direct your focus and energy next month. Our monthly review keeps us from slipping back into "factory robot" mode, where we're just plugging away at the same things without checking in to see if we still actually *want* to do these things, or if we need to change our pace a little, or if we need to add in new weekly small steps to take.

For example, in the sample client's case, let's say she finished writing her outline in one month instead of three. Now, this next month, she may want to add more steps to her "creative" column, such as "write the first page of my novel" as her goal for next month.

Or, alternatively, let's say that now that she's done with her outline, she decides she wants to take a break from writing for a little while. She can therefore swap out her writing column for a new goal she wants to work on that month; in this case, she decides to work on "house organization" projects.

Her new columns for the upcoming month will now look like this:

- **Column One:** College: Study for final exam this month

- **Column Two:** House Organization: Clean up living room and rearrange desk space

- **Column Three:** Self-Care: Meditate, journal, or walk each day

Each month is a chance for you to reflect upon what you just accomplished and what you would like to change going forward to help keep things flowing for you.

Swapping Out Columns

When doing our monthly reviews, we may discover that we haven't been able to move forward with a particular column at all, and this can sometimes be an internal cue that we need to investigate if we still want to continue to work on this specific goal going forward.

> *When procrastination sets in,*
> *self-investigation can begin.*

Stalling out at the starting line happens to all of us sometimes. We change, we grow, and our lives change and grow. We can review and adjust our goal columns as needed, so long as we're consistently taking stock of what's happening with them each month and being honest with ourselves about what we would like to change.

Instead of seeing "stalling out" through a harsh and critical lens, it can be helpful to look at it through a *self-kindness mindset* instead.

Ask yourself:

- *Do I still actually want to achieve this goal?*

- *If so, how can I make this goal easier on myself to start?*

- *If I don't want to do it, what goal will feel more meaningful for me to work on this month, and can I allow myself to swap out my column?*

One client was trying to begin writing a script for a few months and she just couldn't get herself to move forward with it. Even when she made her first step even easier, which was just to brainstorm ideas for it on paper, she said she was "still avoiding doing it" and couldn't get herself to write down any ideas at all.

At our monthly review, I asked her if she wanted to continue with the goal or swap it out with another one that she might like to focus on more instead.

"Yes, I think I want to swap it out," she said with a sigh of relief, "Now that I hear you asking me that, I can admit to myself out loud that I don't really want to do this script anymore. I think this film is an old goal I've been clinging to, back from in college. I think I need to update my goal to where I'm at now, which is that I would like to try relaxing after work by writing songs at the piano instead of trying to work on the script idea anymore."

From this point on, we swapped out her goal column and called it "Music" instead, and suddenly, she was speeding down that column easily with newfound energy and inspiration.

Sometimes, the reason you're feeling stuck is that your goal isn't reflecting who you are *now* and what you actually want to do during this stretch of time. We need to periodically review and update our goals and our vision of what we see ourselves doing now in order to make them reflect where we are in the present moment.

Ask yourself:
Am I hanging onto any outdated goals from a different time in the past?

What goals might need an update to reflect what I'm interested in now instead?

Acknowledge Your Progress

The **End of Month Review** is also a chance for you to emotionally acknowledge the fact that you've made some progress since last month. Did you take a few steps forward? Give yourself some credit and a well-earned pat on the back. You did it! You moved things forward, one step at a time.

Allow yourself to feel proud of yourself at the end of each month for anything that you moved forward even a little bit. The more you practice feeling proud of any small steps you've taken, the more you will be able to feel proud of all the big leaps forward you eventually take as well!

At the end of the month, you can also reflect upon your journey by asking yourself these questions and writing out the answers:

- *What did I do this month that I feel really proud of?*

- *What inspired me this month?*

- *Where did I get stuck this month?*

- *What did I learn this month?*

- *What small step am I glad that I took this month?*

- *What's one encouraging thing I can tell myself going forward?*

Roadblocks and Rest Breaks

After using this goals map for many years, I've learned that there will often be times where things naturally come to a stop on a goal column. For example, on my column called "Therapy," I find there are certain months when the majority of my clients will decide to go on vacation all at once. Or on my other column called "Writing," I'll sometimes find myself waiting for weeks on end to receive notes or feedback.

This is often how our goals work; we often feel stuck, waiting for more information, waiting for collaborators, waiting for answers from people, or just waiting for things to pick up again.

Instead of getting restless during these slower times, I've learned to jump over to my *self-care column* and focus my attention on these goals instead. I start taking more daily walks; I remember to journal more. I catch up on interesting books I've been wanting to read, and I plan more things to do with my family or friends. Sometimes, when one column slows down for a long stretch, you can start taking a small step on another column that you want to give your attention to.

This can be a beneficial way to keep the various areas of your life feeling balanced. We may already do these things unconsciously;

however, learning to switch columns *consciously* can help us feel more empowered. Essentially, you're telling yourself, *"While I can't control some things, I can control where I put my focus and attention next."*

You get to decide what to do with your own energy. What will you choose to focus on next?

Take a Real Break

You may also find that after very busy periods when you've been racing down multiple columns at once, you may need to pause and take a *real break* from everything. This means putting your goals map aside for a little while and just finding the flow of life without planning too far ahead.

Downtime is truly important because it helps our brains and bodies reset. Sometimes, during downtime and breaks is when solutions, insight, and clarity will often appear like magic. Have you ever felt so stuck on something that you decided to get up and go for a walk, and then, halfway through your walk, the solution to your problem just popped into your head? This is because you finally allowed the stress to fully come down a notch, and your brain was able to access its own problem-solving abilities as a result.

Brain Boost:

When we're resting during what we call "downtime," our brains aren't resting at all. Our brains shift into using their "default mode network," which helps us solve problems and retain memories. In this way, our brains are still being productive during periods of rest.

According to Ferris Jabr in his article "Why Downtime Is So Important":

"Downtime replenishes the brain's stores of attention and motivation, encourages productivity and creativity, and is essential to both achieve our highest levels of performance and simply form stable memories in everyday life. A wandering mind unsticks us in time so that we can learn from the past and plan for the future. Moments of respite may even be necessary to keep one's moral compass in working order and maintain a sense of self." (Jabr, F., 2013)

When we finally give our brains enough time to fully unwind, new inspiration and new ideas tend to pop in like friendly visitors who have just been waiting around for any open space to stop by and say hello.

What are some internal signs that you might need more downtime, relaxation, and breaks?

If you're starting to feel really overwhelmed, if you're feeling stressed out for long periods of time, if doing things just isn't feeling fun anymore, or if you're feeling physically, emotionally, or mentally burnt out, these all might be *internal cues* that it's time to take a real break and step away from your goals for a little while.

And then, when you finally get enough rest and let yourself fully reset, you'll naturally feel that energy and inspiration start to kick in again for you. You'll know when this happens because you'll feel excited about setting goals again.

Listen to your brain and body. You really can't do anything without them!

Chapter Two

Creating Calm: Self-Care Is Nonnegotiable

Damage Control Is Not Self-Care

If you've spent years trapped inside of a *toxic productivity mindset*, then you've probably learned to see self-care as *damage control*, rather than as taking care of yourself each day. "Damage control" means that you have worked so hard for so long that you're currently feeling broken, exhausted, emotionally wonky, burnt out, and completely drained, and now you have to face the actual physical, mental, and emotional consequences of this situation.

What does this look like? In an extreme case such as mine, you wind up in the emergency room because you did not listen to what your brain and body were telling you for months on end! In a less extreme case, you might think, *"I'll just relax when I finally take my summer vacation in two months,"* or *"I'm going to push through all this work and then catch up with rest on Sunday* afternoon," or "When I finally get a new job, I'll get things back in balance again."

Even on a smaller day-to-day basis, it might look like, "I'm just going to skip lunches this week because I have so much to catch up on doing," or "It's going to be a really rough month, but I'll catch up on sleep next month instead."

This "storing up self-care points" system does not work out so well for us in reality. We can't just store up life energy "hearts" like we would in a video game and then click on a button to use them whenever our game character has fallen over from exhaustion mid-adventure! We can't instantly restore ourselves after months and months of doing damage to our bodies. It's going to take some real time to get ourselves back in balance, and making self-care a daily priority is how we can help ourselves start to recover.

Self-Care vs. Treats

In addition to associating self-care with "damage control," I have also noticed that when the term "self-care" is mentioned to people, these types of images tend to pop into their heads: vacations, spa visits, going on retreats, buying stuff, travel plans, treating themselves to a fancy meal, and so forth.

All of these things can replenish you once in a while, but they're more like treats and rewards as opposed to daily self-care, because you can't do these things all the time when your stress is starting to rise throughout the day. Daily self-care practices should be things we can do consistently, easily, and without too much planning.

Our self-care should include activities that actively bring our stress down in small notches throughout the day.

Ask yourself: What things would I consider to be daily self-care vs. treats and rewards?

Let's look at one client's list:

Daily Self-Care:	Treats/Rewards:
A few yoga stretches	Going to a yoga retreat
Breathwork meditation	Going to the spa
Knitting or other crafts	Visiting a museum
Sitting outside in the garden	Going on a camping trip

You can see from this client's two columns that her "daily self-care" list included things she could do easily on her own, without much expense.

Now, let's look at the same client's list for **Daily Self-Care vs. Damage Control**. I asked her to describe how doing the self-care activities on the left side column helps her avoid having to do damage control later on the right side.

Daily Self-Care:	Avoiding Damage Control Later:
Regular stretching	Regular stretching keeps my neck from cramping up so I don't have to visit the chiropractor as often. When I stretch each week, I have less back pain.
Breathwork meditation	When I practice deep breathing more often, I have noticed I don't get as anxious, especially if I remember to do it while I'm answering work emails.
Knitting or other crafts	Doing crafts with my hands often helps bring my stress down when I am watching TV. I have less anxiety at night when I spend the evening knitting or doing craft projects. It is a relaxing way to direct my restless energy instead of turning it into anxious thinking.
Sitting outside in the garden	Remembering to step outside into my garden keeps me from getting burned out from working on my computer all day. When I step outside and look around, it helps me get perspective on things.

How might this apply to you?

Make It Nonnegotiable

An actress client was seeing me to work on anxiety and burnout she was feeling while on tour with a show. We had been working on ways she could find her calm backstage, in what she called "really stressful and chaotic environments where there is nowhere to just bring the anxiety down without being interrupted every few minutes."

We had already established a nightly self-care routine for when she was not on tour, where she would write in her journal, put on headphones to listen to guided meditations, and practice letting go of her worries from that day. It was a set of daily practices that worked really well at home, and one that she had started to look forward to after long days of rehearsals.

"When I've had a long day of rehearsing, just sitting alone with my journal helps me organize my thoughts," she said, "And wearing the headphones makes space inside my head, so I don't get anxious about everything around me when I have them on."

While this routine worked great for her at home, she was having trouble doing any of it when she was on tour, going to different cities and having to "camp out for hours [backstage] in greenrooms." She was having a lot of pre-show anxiety and was finding it difficult to ground herself in places that felt uncomfortable to her.

One session, she joked about how a fellow actor wanted to add "a reclining lazy boy chair" to their "rider list" because they all just needed somewhere to take a nap and get away from the stress of the tour. I asked her what a rider list was, and she explained, "It's a list of requested items that you get in the greenroom, like fancy water bottles or special sandwiches you like. You know, like those nonnegotiable lists big-time celebrities get to make so when they get to the greenroom, the stuff they like is waiting for them. We don't have one like that."

"Maybe you need your own nonnegotiable self-care list—one that you make for yourself for things you want to remember to bring with you," I said, inspired.

"Nonnegotiable self-care. I like that! What would I put on my list?" she inquired. She had never thought to take care of herself in this way.

"Whatever calms you down. Your journal, your coloring pencils, your headphones...whatever has been working for you at home, you would bring those types of things. Make a nonnegotiable self-care kit for yourself," I suggested.

"But can I make it all fit inside the bag I bring backstage?"

"It's nonnegotiable," I laughed.

"Then I'll figure it out!" she laughed.

After the session, she was inspired to create what she described as her "nonnegotiable self-care kit," which was small and easy to fit in her bag. Before each show, she would find a small space in the greenroom to put on her headphones and listen to a guided meditation while drawing in her notebook for half an hour. She found that even taking just a half hour to create this space for herself was helping to calm down her pre-show anxiety quite a bit.

"The new self-care kit is working," she told me a few months later. "When I remember to use it, I manage to carve out some space for myself to bring the stress down a little before the show. It's really simple to do, I just never thought to take care of myself in this way before. I never thought of it as all that important. And now, I just tell myself it's completely nonnegotiable!"

She even found that adopting this new mindset was starting to change what she wanted to do after the shows as well.

"I used to rush around and go out all night after performances, and that would make me so tired and exhausted the next day," she said, "Now I find that sometimes I'm choosing to stay in my hotel room and just let myself recover and rest. I write in my journal or I read my book. It makes me feel like I'm taking care of myself, like I'm not fighting myself and battling my own exhaustion anymore."

Somehow, when you tell people that self-care is *nonnegotiable*, their brains suddenly decide to see it as essential to accomplish. There's no more "I should/would/could" do these things. It becomes: *"I need to do these things, there is no choice except to do them."*

Instead of, *"I can just work through all my breaks to get all these emails done,"* it becomes, *"I need to step away from the computer right now and go for a walk to get some perspective on things."* Instead of, *"I can play with the kids later after I finally finish this work proposal,"* it becomes, *"I'm going to take a quick break and play with the kids now because it cheers me up, makes me smile, and reminds me of the things I value the most."*

Instead of, *"It's okay I'm stressed out because I have a vacation coming up next month where I can get some relaxation in,"* it becomes, *"If I want to really enjoy my vacation next month, I should let myself relax a little each day before then so that I will be in a better place mentally and physically to enjoy it."* Instead of, *"I can push through doing errands on the way home from work even though I'm feeling tired and out of it,"* it becomes, *"I should go home and let myself rest, and then tomorrow morning, I will have so much more energy to get stuff done."*

Seeing things through this new lens will start to change your daily choices, your relationship with *yourself*, and even how you're experiencing time.

We need to remind ourselves that taking care of our brains and bodies is really this important.

In fact, it's nonnegotiable!

The Stress Scale

In order to get stuff done without the stress, it's useful to figure out just how much stress we're experiencing right now. "Stress" is one of those terms we throw around a lot, but in actuality, I have found that most people don't really think about it very much until it's so very high that they can't *not* think about it. In other words, we tend to wait until we're completely losing it with stress before we even admit to ourselves that we're feeling any of it at all!

As a matter of fact, stress is a normal thing we're experiencing all day long, and our stress levels go up and down all the time. You can think of it like this:

| 1 | 2 | 3 | 4 | 5 | 6 | 7 | 8 | 9 | 10 |

Lowest   Highest
Stress   Stress

This maps a range of stress with different notches that can feel very different for different people. On the low end near "1," you feel little to no stress. On the "10" side, you experience a very high level of stress.

Many people may only realize they're stressed out when they're on the higher end of the scale. However, there are often internal cues you can start to become more aware of that your stress is climbing up one small notch at a time. And if you can learn what these internal and external **signs of stress** look like for you, you'll be able to catch them and address the sources of stress *before* you get to the very high end of the scale.

Ask yourself:
What internal cues do you feel when stress is rising in your brain and body?

What external signs do others notice about you when your stress level is getting higher?

Let's look at one client's answers:

When I start to feel a high level of stress, I...

Internal Signs	External Signs
I get headaches.	I start losing my sense of humor and I'm grumpy.
I can't stop worrying.	I can't find things like my keys and phone.
I have a lot of trouble focusing.	I am late for appointments and meetings.
I feel worn out but won't let myself rest.	I want to isolate and be on my own too much.

What are your internal and external signs of stress?

The Tipping Point

In most everyday situations, our stress is like a slow simmer that starts to build and build until it eventually boils over. The trick is to identify the causes of your stress before you reach the *tipping point* when stress hormones such as cortisol and adrenaline begin to flood your brain and body, because after that point, it becomes harder and harder to physically calm yourself down.

What number on the scale might be a tipping point for you? As an example, most people will say it's a 7 or 8 on their scale, and that if they pass that point, they will often just shoot up to a 10 very quickly. Other people might say their tipping point is more of a 6 on the scale, because even this lower level starts to feel uncomfortable to them.

When we can identify what our own *tipping point* feels like in our own brain and body, we start to more intentionally catch our own stress as it's rising each day.

What might your tipping point be on the above scale? What are some internal and external signs that you're reaching that point? How would someone observing you know that you were at your tipping point?

Some examples of tipping point signs I tend to hear from clients include: Becoming grumpy, wanting to withdraw and isolate, taking things too personally, becoming overly sensitive to noises or other sensory stimuli around them, feeling overwhelmed, snapping at loved ones, not knowing what task to do next, not taking any breaks, forgetting to stop working, getting overly busy with things they don't need to do, or losing their sense of humor completely.

What does it look like for you? It's different for every single person.

Most of us are experiencing a lot of stress rising throughout our day. And stress can negatively impact our immune systems, it can impact our daily sleep, it can mess up our digestion, it can cause us to have body tension and headaches, and it can raise our blood pressure, according to multiple studies done over the last decade (Ross, S. 2020). Chronic stress can even shrink our brains!

Brain Boost:

Neuroscientist Amy Arsten claims that experiencing chronic stress can actually shrink parts of your brain: "One of the most striking (effects) is thinning of the gray matter of an area of the brain called the prefrontal cortex," Arnsten states. "It's a double whammy. At the same time the prefrontal cortex is getting weaker and more primitive, the brain circuits that generate emotion like fear are getting stronger. You start seeing the world as harmful even when it's not." (Lamotte, S., CNN Health)

This is why it's so important to identify and acknowledge our own stress levels, so that we can take deliberate steps to take care of ourselves and bring the stress down, a little at a time.

Using the Scale

What do each of these notches on the scale feel like to your brain and body when you experience them? How is a 6 different than a 7, or a 2 different from a 3? All of these various stress levels look different on different people.

Here is an example of one client's **Stress Scale**:

1. *Calm/mellow/relaxed.*

2. *Calm but getting busier with more things.*

3. *Busier, starting to rush around more, but still feeling okay overall.*

4. *Feeling low levels of stress, but able to push stressful thoughts aside.*

5. *Feeling more stressful thoughts popping in, feeling more "intense," and having a little trouble relaxing after work and on weekends.*

6. *Getting pulled in many directions, starting to feel some tension about what to do next.*

7. *Starting to have more anxiety and stressful thoughts, getting grumpier and more short-tempered with people around me.*

8. **Tipping Point:** *Really stressed out, nothing feels fun to do, little things really bother me that don't usually bother me at all. Tension in neck, headaches.*

9. *Emotionally drained and overwhelmed, can't make decisions anymore.*

10. *Freaking out. I feel totally shut down. I feel frozen and stuck. I can't remember how to calm down, and I can't decide what to do next.*

Now, it's your turn. What do these stress levels look like on you?

Write out what the different levels of stress feel like to you, with 1 being the lowest and 10 the highest, then circle your **tipping point** number:

1.

2.

3.

4.

5.

6.

7.

8.

9.

10.

So, what can you do, when you find yourself at your *tipping point*? Write down a few activities that you can do that can bring your stress down, one notch at a time.

Write out a self-care activity you can do for each notch of the scale, starting with what you can do when you're calmer (1-5) vs. different self-care activities that might work when you are higher on the scale (6-10).

1.

2.

3.

4.

5.

6.

7.

8.

9.

10.

It's helpful to remember that stress doesn't just turn off like a light switch. We can't go from a 10 down to a 1 instantly. We have to bring our stress down one level at a time, by purposefully choosing to take actions that calm us down. We have to wait for the cortisol and adrenaline to subside, which can sometimes take *several hours* to happen, and then we also have to avoid respiking our stress levels up to the high end of the scale during this stretch of time.

In other words, we have to let ourselves *fully reset.*

A lot of the time, we may be taking breaks at set times on the clock, but our stress level stays exactly the same throughout the break. Going forward, a *real break* means that you are actively taking steps to lower your stress a notch on your scale. Maybe this means stepping away from your computer, going for a walk, and letting your mind wander for a few minutes. Maybe this means doing some deep breathing or doodling in your notebook until you feel a little relief.

Whatever self-care activities you choose to engage in, make sure you are actually giving your brain and body a *real* break, instead of just calling it one!

When Stress Signs Are Subtle

I work with many people who work in professions where they have to maintain their composure all day long, such as CEOs, therapists, doctors, performers, directors, and teachers. They learn to wear a "mask of calm" at work, because they have to, it's part of their jobs. This doesn't mean they *aren't* getting stressed out, it just means that the stress is being repressed and so it's getting shoved down beneath the surface on a regular basis.

While this is often necessary for them to be able to do their jobs, the problem is that, at home, it might not be so obvious to loved ones that they are under any stress at all because they aren't showing any obvious physical signs of it. And then, when they finally do erupt into visible stress, it can really shock and surprise the people around them. This divide between the stress people are *feeling* and the stress people are visibly *showing* can sometimes cause confusion and conflict with others.

Do you have to wear a "mask of calm" all day? And do you sometimes mask your own level of stress from yourself? Do you often tell yourself, "I'm fine!" when you're not really feeling that "fine" at all?

If this is the case for you, learning to use the stress scale can help you identify where your stress levels really are more of the time.

Using the Scale to Communicate

Having an easy way to express to others that our stress is rising on the scale can become a useful tool for effectively communicating our needs.

One client learned to tell his wife that his stress was at level "8" by just saying, "I'm at an 8!" Then she knew to not take his mood as personally. "It's helped our relationship a lot," he explained in a session, "because before, she never knew how high my stress actually was. I have to hide it at work because I have to manage many people and keep my calm all day long. Now, I can tell her in a simple statement that I'm high on my scale, and we no longer have so many misunderstandings. She knows to give me space until I can bring my stress down a little. She's also started telling me when she's feeling her stress rise on the scale too, and I've learned that I need to step in and help her out more then."

In this way, we can learn to tell people how high our stress levels are, and we can learn to listen more effectively when other people tell us about theirs as well. We often assume other people aren't stressed out at all, but this may not be true; in fact, I'd argue that most people are pretty high up on their stress scales these days. However, since we all have different ways of showing our stress, we won't really know what level of stress someone else is experiencing unless we ask them.

Using the **Stress Scale** is an easy way to start developing a better awareness of our own emotional states and to learn to tell each other what we're experiencing in the moment. When we can learn to recognize the subtle signs of our daily stress rising, we can take more proactive steps to bring our stress down when it's on the lower end of the scale, rather than doing damage control after we've already exceeded level 10.

How Stress Makes Us Stuck

Have you ever wondered why on certain days it's impossible to pick what outfit to wear, what lunch to eat, or what sentence to type in an email, while on other days, these things may only take you thirty seconds to complete? Why do tiny daily tasks sometimes feel so arduous and challenging for us to do?

A simple answer: You're probably more stressed out than you think! As a result, your brain is likely shutting down your executive functioning skills, including your ability to make decisions, prioritize actions, and find the first step forward with tasks.

Feeling high levels of stress each day can impair our executive functions, which are entirely necessary for getting things done.

Our executive functions include:

- **Task Initiation:** Our ability to get started on things we need to do and figure out what the first step forward is.

- **Organization:** How we sort, arrange, and organize tasks.

- **Cognitive Flexibility:** Our ability to adjust to the unexpected, make new decisions, and rearrange priorities based on new information we receive.

- **Working Memory:** How we keep track of what we need to do and remember all the pieces of projects we need to complete.

- **Impulse Control:** Being able to think before we act and being able to assess the outcome of our actions is crucial to managing our time effectively.

- **Self-Monitoring:** Our ability to track our own progress on a project and figure out how many steps are left to complete it.

- **Emotional Control:** When we get tipped over into emotions like frustration, anxiety, anger, and overwhelm, how quickly can we find our way back to calm again? Regulating our emotions is a crucial part of being able to access all of our other executive functions.

When our prefrontal cortex becomes "frozen" from stress, our executive functioning can suffer. According to a Temple University study, when people experience high levels of stress and overwhelm, the prefrontal cortex "goes dark" on the MRI, which means that activity in that region of the brain freezes up temporarily while the stress is happening.

Brain Boost:

When we become stressed out, our prefrontal cortex, which controls our executive functions, can become impaired. According to Michael Vaughan, author of the *Entrepreneur Magazine* article "Know Your Limits, Your Brain Can Only Take So Much," Temple University scientists noticed suspended activity in the prefrontal cortex area on MRI scans when participants became overwhelmed and stressed out with information. This caused the participants to make "bad choices because the brain region responsible for smart decision making has essentially left the premises." (Vaughan, 2014.)

In other words, stress can make our brains feel "instantly jammed up;" but by taking the time to deliberately calm ourselves down, we can access our executive functioning skills again.

This is why regulating our stress is so very important to do, and why finding our calm really does help us get stuff done.

Your Capacity for Calm

When we're experiencing stress, our *fight-or-flight* sympathetic nervous system is triggered. This sends cortisol and adrenaline pumping into our systems and engages our amygdala, ramping up our feelings of fear and vigilance to a state of full alert. This can raise our heart rate, increase our blood glucose, and quicken our breath. When we're in this fight-or-flight mode, it becomes very difficult to access the more logical parts of our brains that can help us organize our thoughts, remember things, or make decisions. In other words, our brains have been completely hijacked by our amygdala and our sympathetic nervous system.

On the other side of things, our parasympathetic nervous system (PNS) controls our body's "rest and digest" functions and produces a very calming and relaxing effect on the body. It lowers our heart rate, instigates digestion, and resets us from the harsh effects of the sympathetic nervous system.

Somatic grounding techniques seek to activate our parasympathetic nervous system through breathwork, movement, mindfulness, or otherwise using our senses in a relaxing way. We're trying to intentionally trigger the "rest and digest" mode to deactivate the fight-or-flight reaction so that we can calm our brains and bodies down in the moment.

By learning more ways to ground ourselves in calmness more regularly, we're expanding our capacity to feel calm, a little bit at a time.

One effective way I've found to bring my stress down quickly when I start to reach my tipping point is to do simple breathwork exercises for a few minutes in a row. Deep breathing is free, it only takes a couple minutes to do, and most of the time, other people won't notice that you're doing it. This is why breathing exercises are taught to first responders such as firefighters, emergency room doctors, nurses, and counselors to help them manage their stress during crisis situations. Even pilots and flight attendants are sometimes taught *Box Breathing* as a way to handle mid-air crisis situations. But it can also work for you in non-crisis situations, too. You can use something like Box Breathing when you're loading the dishwasher, driving through rush-hour traffic, or trying to get through that endless staff meeting.

A quick note on breathwork: It doesn't work in the same way for everyone. Our nervous systems are all very diverse, and we are wired in different ways. While deep breathing works really well for many people, there are certain people who won't respond in a relaxing way to it; in fact, it might make them feel anxious or tense at first.

Somatic exercises work in different ways and at different speeds for different people. It took me many months of practicing breathwork to even feel any of its relaxing effects, and I really struggled with learning how to deeply exhale when I first tried it. Listen to what your body is telling you, and then adjust accordingly. Figure out what works to calm your own nervous system down in small increments. It can also be helpful to work with a therapist, instructor, or another practitioner who specializes in somatic-based exercises or mindfulness if you want to explore any of these tools in more depth to find the ones that will work best for you.

Box Breathing

Box Breathing is a simple breathing exercise developed by Mark Divine, a Navy Seal, that helps you control your breath by picturing your breath traveling around a square. A study done in 2017 showed that diaphragmatic breathing such as what you do during Box Breathing "significantly" lowered participants' cortisol levels after only fifteen minutes of doing it. (Ma, Xiu, Front. Psychol., 05 June 2017)

You can visualize Box Breathing like this:

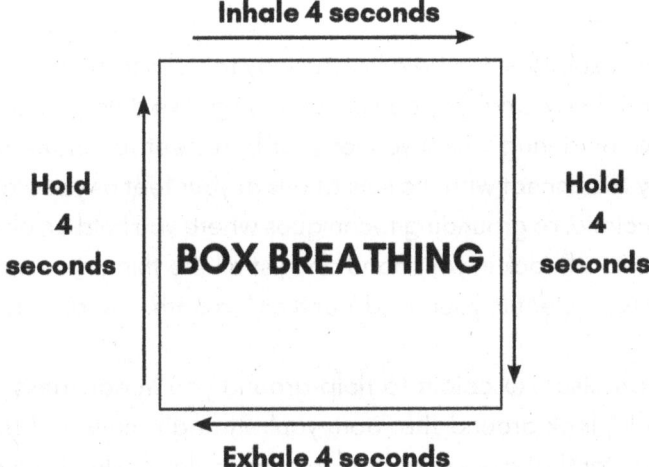

Breathe in for four seconds, hold for four seconds, breathe out for four seconds, and hold for four seconds. For many people, it helps to count the numbers in your head so that you purposefully slow down your breath.

An easy place to start practicing breathing techniques is just to let out a sigh when you feel the stress start to build up. Let that exhale out with a whoosh of breath, and try to drop the tension in your shoulders as you do it. See if this helps reduce the stress a little bit for you.

Grounding Techniques

Sometimes, our brains feel like they're floating away on a thought cloud, drifting away into stress, anxiety and worries, and we can easily forget about our bodies down below. By checking in with our bodies throughout the day, we can find our sense of alignment and tap into our own calm inner strength again. We can bring our brains back home to our bodies in this way.

Sensory exercises can be a helpful way to deliberately check in with your body, and they can include things like doing a walking meditation during which you let your bare feet touch the floor and try to connect with the sensations of your feet as you walk in a slow circle, or grounding techniques where you hold an object like a smooth rock in your hand and list all the things you notice about the object in your mind (such as "smooth, round, gray").

You can also use colors to help ground you in calmness. For example, look around the room you're in right now and try to find a color that makes you feel relaxed, calm, or simply neutral and just focus your attention on it for a little while. If you want to take a few long deep breaths while you're doing this, it may even help you calm down faster. Or pick up a marker in a color that you like and fill up a whole blank page with it until you start to feel a little more relaxed.

Listening to relaxing music, including binaural beats in music, as well as *white, pink or brown noise* or other soothing sounds also helps many people center themselves when they start to feel overwhelmed. You can start to proactively use music as a calming tool by planning out soothing playlists for stressful times of day. For instance, on your long commute home from work, what music can you play that will make you feel calm and relaxed? Repeat this same calming playlist every day on your way home, and watch how your brain starts to expect and crave it after a little while.

Some people respond well to using touch as a grounding sense. The *Butterfly Hug,* which is used by many *EMDR* therapists, involves crossing your arms over your chest and alternating tapping your hands on your shoulders (left, right, left, right) over and over again until you start to calm down a little. You can also put your hands on your knees if you're sitting down and alternate tapping on your legs, too. It's a self-soothing technique that provides *bilateral stimulation*, which often helps pull people out of their stressful thoughts and back into the present moment again.

Other people prefer to use an aroma as a sensory grounding tool, since smell is one of our most powerful senses. Just by our smelling a particular scent that we associate with happy emotions from a specific time, our brains can often reproduce these emotions for us to experience almost instantly, as if the scent was a magical portal back to that specific memory.

Brain Boost:

Smells have direct access through the olfactory bulb straight to our limbic system, which triggers regions in the brain related to emotions and memory. Dr. Rachel Herz reported in the journal *Brain Sciences*, "Odors that evoke positive autobiographical memories have the potential to increase positive emotions, decrease negative mood states, disrupt cravings, and reduce physiological indices of stress, including systemic markers of inflammation." (Herz, R. 2016) Our sense of smell is so powerful that even if you just think about a smell it can instantly evoke memories of it. Try it right now—think of a smell you like, and see if you can feel the feelings related to it.

Ask yourself:

What smells make me feel happy?

What types of sounds calm me down?

What colors make me feel calm or relaxed?

What visuals might work to help me bring my stress down?

What is an object that might feel calming to hold?

By connecting with our senses more intentionally, we can start to feel more aligned with what's happening in our bodies in the present moment, which helps us find our inner strength again.

Your Tipping Point Hours

Many people find that late afternoons tend to be their *tipping point hours*, the time when stress runs high after working all day. If this is the case for you, what will you plan to do differently in the late afternoon from now on? Can you take a pause to go for a walk outside? Can you put on a relaxing playlist for the drive home? Can you remember to take some of those long deep breaths in and out each day at four in the afternoon? Can you give yourself a little *calm buffer break* by listening to a guided meditation before dinner to bring the stress down a little?

Which times of day does your stress tend to reach the tipping point?

What can you plan to do to actively bring your stress down during these times?

When are your *tipping point* hours?

The Calm Zone

The truth is, most of us get more regular practice at feeling stressed out than we do at feeling calm. When I ask people to fill out the stress scale, they will often tell me that they "can't remember what a 1 on the scale even feels like," or "It's been so long since I've felt under a 5, I can't really identify it," or "If I ever get below a 3, I never stay there for very long."

Let's call all the numbers below 5 our *calm zone* and start to think about how to let ourselves visit this state of being more frequently throughout the week to balance things out. In this way, we're beginning to learn to expand our *capacity to feel calm.*

Think about this right now. What would the *lack* of stress feel like to you? Try to remember a past time when you felt very low on your stress scale. Where were you and what were you doing? Hold onto a specific image that represents this calm and peaceful time. Now, whenever you think of this image, try to feel the calm feelings you have associated with it. A few times each day, bring this *calm image* to the forefront of your mind and practice feeling peaceful for a minute or two.

We can learn to get comfortable with what calm feels like in tiny moments and slowly stretch out our *calm capacity* over time.

> *Practice the feelings you want to feel, and you will be able to feel them more often.*

What are some tiny ways you can practice visiting your *calm zone* today? Even if it's only for a few minutes, those few minutes can make a big difference to your brain and body. Those few minutes may even keep you from reaching your tipping point by the end of this day.

> *Taking a few minutes to find your calm will naturally help you get stuff done.*

Sometimes you have to deliberately slow down to finish things faster. And sometimes you have to stop being so busy in order to stop feeling so stuck. When we slow down on purpose and bring down our stress intentionally, time often seems to stretch to suit our needs.

Protecting Your Calm

What kinds of things tend to pull you out of calmness? How do you lose your balance in this way? Take out a piece of paper and draw a square, then label it: Calm Zone.

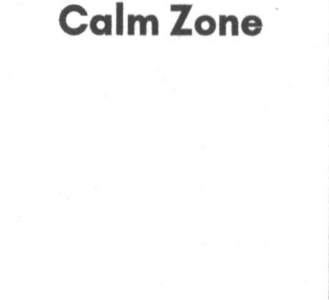

What things might be outside of the walls of this square that tend to take away your calm? Write these things out on the outside perimeters of the square. Here's an example from one client:

	Calm Zone	
Trying to micro-manage projects when I can delegate more tasks		Going to too many social things on the weekends
Checking work messages at night before bed		Not planning out errands I need to do in advance and trying to do too many all on same day

Now, what can we write in the middle section to remind ourselves to stay in our *calm zone* more regularly? Here is the same client's drawing:

Calm Zone

Trying to micro-manage projects when I can delegate more tasks	Put my phone away for a few hours at night	Going to too many social things on the weekends
Checking work messages at night before bed	Plan out my time on the weekends to do more things I find relaxing and calm	Not planning out errands I need to do in advance and trying to do too many all on same day
	Order groceries online to save time on weeknds	

What would go inside and outside of your square?

Becoming Mindful About Mind Chatter

In addition to considering external messages and factors that tend to take away our calm, it's also helpful to consider all the ways we tend to take it away from *ourselves*. Sometimes, when we're finally able to relax a little, our brains will stir up internal drama with a big wave of overly critical mind chatter.

When things are calm, do you start to review all of your past mistakes? Do you start to yell at yourself about all of the unfinished items on your to-do list? Do you say to yourself, *"You shouldn't be sitting here relaxing, you have too much to do!"* Do you beat yourself up, talk to yourself in really harsh ways, or make yourself feel "bad" about "not being productive"?

Brain Boost:

After conducting a two-week study where students were asked to record all of their thoughts in a "brutally honest" style, Dr. Raj Raghunathan observed that daily "'mental chatter,' so to speak—is mostly (up to 70 percent) negative, a phenomenon that could be referred to as negativity dominance." He concluded: "Deep down, it turns out that people are much more self-critical, pessimistic, and fearful than they let out in their conscious thoughts" (Raghunathan, 2013).

Where does this type of harsh self-talk come from? When you were younger, what messages did you hear about relaxing or being "lazy"? What messages did you receive about being productive or staying "busy"? Were you around adults who were always rushing around because they never knew how to slow down, relax, or really rest for any length of time?

Ask yourself: What did I learn growing up from the adults around me about being calm or about being busy?

Our culture's push toward chronic *busyness* often starts really early. I don't know about where you live, but here in Los Angeles, it's pretty common for kids to spend most of their free time being rushed around to extracurricular activities, and for parents to spend most of their spare time driving kids around from one thing to the next, often enduring endless gridlock traffic.

Sometimes when I work with parents who are feeling exhausted, I ask them to consider that if *they're* feeling burnt out from constant activities each week, how might their *kids* be feeling? We often assume kids have endless amounts of energy, but they get exhausted and burned out just like the rest of us do. Their bodies and minds are still growing (which is exhausting in and of itself), and they're constantly having to learn new things, talk to new people, learn new skills, learn new rules, adapt to new environments, and transition between different places; and sometimes, depending on their personalities, all of these things can feel very overwhelming for them to do. By the end of the week, is it any wonder that our kids are melting down or at least acting a little grumpy?

If you're noticing that you and your family members are stressed out, exhausted, or drained on a frequent basis, it can be helpful to take stock of where everyone is at on their own *stress scales.*

We can teach our family members to communicate their stress using the scale and ask them to give us a rating readout when we sense the stress is running high.

And then, we can practice cognitive flexibility by making regular adjustments to our schedules based upon everyone's general well-being needs each week. Can you cut back on a few activities to slow down the pace on certain days of the week? Can you skip doing a few things this weekend to bring the stress down a little for everyone?

After all, when our kids grow up, we want them to know how to relax, unwind, and fully reset, just like we also want them to learn skills and participate in all the wonderful pursuits that they find fulfilling. In other words, we want them to find their own unique sense of balance in their lives.

We can show them how to do this by finding our own sense of balance and by adjusting things on a regular basis to maintain it.

Drawing Lines with Time

Often, the reason we're overbooking ourselves is because we're getting stuck in chronic people-pleasing mode, where we are trying to keep everyone around us happy, all of the time. It's an impossible trap we put ourselves in, because we can't really control other peoples' emotions, and trying to keep everyone else "happy" often comes at the expense of our own mental, physical, and emotional well-being.

Transforming this pattern starts with getting really honest with yourself about how stressed out and exhausted you're currently feeling. Fully accept where you are right now instead of chronically trying to push through things to keep everyone happy, or telling yourself you're "fine" when you're running high on stress and low on energy. Acknowledge what your brain and body are feeling in this moment. Then, make the tiny decision that it's important for you to get back in balance again by establishing boundaries to protect your time.

Setting boundaries can feel uncomfortable at first, but it gets easier the more you practice doing it. At first, when you turn down invitations or other obligations to protect your time and well-being, you may feel really guilty afterward because you're breaking an old pattern that you may have been practicing for many years. In these moments of true discomfort, it's helpful to remind yourself that it only feels like this because it's new and different. It won't feel uncomfortable in this way forever, it just takes a little consistent practice over time.

When it comes to setting time boundaries, state things in the simplest way you can think of, and try to avoid backpedaling or overexplaining too much, as this tends to confuse the listener. Certain people around you may not have the healthiest time boundaries themselves, and so it might be uncomfortable for them to see you practicing doing something that feels different to them at first. Be consistent with what you're saying, and they will adjust, you will adjust, and over time, you will find that it's starting to feel much easier for you to do.

Here are some soothing things you can tell yourself as you practice setting time boundaries:

- *"I am learning to be kinder to myself, one step a time."*

- *"Taking care of my brain and body is nonnegotiable from now on. I can let myself take a real break and pull back from things until I'm fully recharged again."*

- *"Being kinder to myself will allow me to be much kinder to other people, and I will have much more to give if I let myself reset first."*

- *"By getting enough rest and taking a step back, I can get more perspective on things and figure out what I really want to do with my time going forward."*

Remember: By rating everyone else's demands and needs as higher in priority on our to-do list, we're essentially moving our own needs further and further down. While this is sometimes necessary to do in certain circumstances, we can't treat ourselves as the last on our own list all of the time.

Shifting Your Self-Talk

If you catch your brain stirring up the drama with harsh and overly critical mind chatter during downtime, try to notice it a little more intentionally, but from a distance, like you're an observer watching it play out. When we observe our thoughts, our thoughts will naturally start to change.

We can call out and label this *harsh mind chatter* a little more regularly when it happens, and then we can ask ourselves, *"Am I trying to take away my own calm right now? Can I allow myself to stay here for a little while instead?"*

Here are some examples of calming phrases you might start to introduce into your self-talk stream instead:

- *"I can allow myself to take a break right now. I can be kind to myself in this way."*

- *"I don't have to do anything right now. I can really allow myself some space to feel calmness for a little while."*

- *"If I let myself rest and reset, everything will feel much easier for me to do."*

- *"Downtime is beneficial for my brain and body as it helps me find balance and clarity."*

- *"I can go at my own pace. I can slow down when I need to."*

- *"Relaxing is just as important as doing things. I'm finding my own balance right now."*

- *"I'm learning to see slowing down as a way I can be kinder to myself."*

Imagine how you would talk to a friend about taking breaks and letting themselves reset when they really needed to. How would you soothe them, encourage them, and show them a little support?

Then, start to talk to yourself as though you are *your own friend.* After all, wouldn't you like to be, from now on?

Addicted to Adrenaline

If we've been caught up in a *toxic productivity mindset* for most of our adult lives, we've probably been functioning close to our tipping point on the stress scale on a daily basis. As a result, we may have also accidentally become psychologically addicted to the sensation of what adrenaline feels like in our bodies, since adrenaline tends to give us an extra boost of energy.

Brain Boost:

In addition to adrenaline and cortisol, the body releases dopamine when it's under stress, and dopamine gives us a feeling of *reward*. According to Dr. Debbie Sorensen, the mixture of adrenaline and dopamine can be "as addictive as drugs" to some (Smith, M., 2023). We may therefore find ourselves craving both the energy boost of adrenaline and the rewarding feeling of dopamine, and we may keep ourselves *chronically busy and stressed* to get more of it.

Many people are so used to living with the "go-go-go" feeling that being still almost feels "painfully uncomfortable" to experience, as one client put it.

"When I finally get some time to relax on the weekend," she said, "I wind up planning so much to do that before I know it, I'm rushing around again. I think I struggle with being still for long stretches, and I don't know how to navigate that feeling. I really don't like it!"

If this *adrenaline rush* has become your default setting, then feeling calm will sometimes feel challenging to experience in contrast. It can be helpful to start to rewrite what "calm" feels like to you so that you can learn to associate it with more pleasant feelings instead of pushing it away and avoiding it by default.

Ask yourself, "What words do I currently associate with calm?"

Write out a list of words, noticing if these words have any negative connotations for you.

For example, this was one client's list of word associations with the concept of calmness:

- Boring, restless, uncomfortable, silent, frustrating

When we explored these associations, many of them came from her childhood, where she often felt like she was being "forced" by teachers and parents to "be still and quiet" for "long stretches of time that felt like they went on forever."

However, we can start to gradually shift these associations for ourselves over time. Calm can mean "quiet and stillness," but it doesn't necessarily have to mean these things if you don't want it to. You can decide that it can mean things like: *Peace, awareness, balance, feeling okay, relaxation, happiness, coziness, appreciation,* or other pleasant emotions.

For example, this same client wrote out these new associations that she liked better:

- Okay, neutral, relaxed, in the flow, mellow, coziness

You can redefine what calm means to you on a daily basis. Maybe "calm" means curling up in your favorite chair, sipping tea slowly, and embracing a new cozy feeling you label in your mind. Maybe it means stepping outside before work starts and taking a few deep breaths of morning air. Or maybe it means slowing down when you're going out for a walk and noticing the bright colors of flowers around you a little more deliberately.

When calm starts to feel more comfortable to your brain, your brain will start to crave calmness more of the time.

Give yourself full permission to leave a little more space for the calm to come in.

Invite it in, welcome it with open arms, and see how your whole life begins to change in entirely new ways.

Chapter Three

Design Your Time: Creating Space for Things That Matter

Creating Space

Now that we've created internal space for calmer feelings, how can we create actual space in our schedule each week to get stuff done? Creating space is more than just leaving a few hours free in your calendar to methodically plug in tasks and projects; it's about figuring out what's important and essential to you and then taking steps to protect these things...from *yourself*!

Because the truth is that most of us are crunching our own time, and we don't even know we're doing it.

Brain Boost:

In a study of seven thousand participants, researchers compared how people felt about their time compared to how much time they actually had to do tasks. In their conclusions, they stated, "Those who felt most overworked...largely do it to themselves," and, "Much of the time devoted to paid and unpaid tasks is over and above that which is strictly necessary. In that sense, much of the time pressure that people feel is discretionary and of their own making." (Goodin *et al.* 2004, p.45.) So, a lot of the time, we're making ourselves *feel* like we don't have enough time by taking on much too much to do (including what we didn't necessarily have to do in the first place)!

Here are some common misconceptions people tend to have about their own ability to manage their time:

- They expect themselves to have *unlimited* energy and focus each day

- They expect themselves to complete as many tasks as possible by plugging them into every spare slot in their calendar

- They tend to avoid downtime as it will "derail" them from generating output

Instead, here are some reality-based truths about our own ability to manage our time:

- We have very *limited* amounts of focus and energy each day

- While we can accomplish lots of tasks, each one costs us energy, and some tasks cost us *far more* energy than others

- Downtime is just as important as focus to our brains; we need it to function effectively

- Our brains tend to need a mix of focus, fun, and rest each week to stay balanced

Ask yourself: How much focus, fun, rest, or downtime do I need to feel balanced each week?

Which of these things do I need more of right now?

The Time Wardrobe

Imagine a wardrobe-type closet sitting in a room. When you open the closet, it's jam-packed full of stuff stacked all the way up to the top. Even as you open the doors, things start to topple over and fall out onto you. It's just packed *that* full.

Let's say you decide to go to the store and purchase elaborate systems, racks, baskets, and shelves to organize your closet. After you install all of these things, everything might look orderly for a moment or two. But then, after a few days, your wardrobe closet gradually starts to descend into disarray. Weeks later, when you open your closet, you realize you can't even see the elaborate racks and shelves you just installed because they are completely lost under piles and piles of stuff! Because the simple truth of the matter is that you just have too much stuff in there and no system is really going to work all that well until you address this core issue.

Now, imagine this stuffed wardrobe closet is your *weekly schedule*!

Just like the closet in our example, we're probably stuffing our weekly schedule much too full of tasks, errands, chores, and projects each week. So, in order to get things to work for us in a calmer way, we're going to really need to simplify our time down and stop overextending ourselves on a regular basis. It's about getting more intentional about what you're putting in your schedule and what you're leaving out.

Designing Your Time

For most of us, our work schedule is already taking up a very large chunk of space on our weekly calendar. Our jobs usually fill up eight hours of each day with meetings, projects, and other time-bound activities that are already slotted and scheduled into our time already.

So for now, let's look at the unscheduled time that's *outside of work*, since this time is more open to our efforts to redesign our scheduling, and let's start to think about what we want to create with this space.

How do we want to design our free time this week?

Free Time vs. Focus Time

There are definitely occasions when we should wing it with our time. When we're on vacation, relaxing, or out having fun somewhere, we don't need to proactively figure out what we're doing in every free hour of time. In fact, doing this can be very stressful for us to experience. Instead, during this type of free time, we can just practice being in the moment a little more and letting time flow. Sometimes, we can embrace unscheduled time in our calendar and use it to rest, relax, have fun, and just see what happens next without planning anything at all.

However, I've learned there is a difference between having *free time* and *time to focus* scheduled in your calendar, and it's important to clearly define the differences between the two and separate them out from each other.

Many people often have an unstated idea that there are two types of time: "Work Time" and "Free Time," and it looks something like this:

```
┌──────────────┐  ┌──────────────┐
│              │  │              │
│              │  │              │
│              │  │              │
│    Work      │  │  Free Time   │
│              │  │              │
│              │  │              │
│              │  │              │
└──────────────┘  └──────────────┘
```

But they are usually trying to shove extremely too many things into the "Free Time" box. It's overflowing with errands, tasks, hobbies, family stuff, social activities, exercise, creative projects, and so on. Nothing is sorted in there; they're just trying to wing it each week with this jumbled up messy box of scattered stuff! You can imagine it like this:

```
┌──────────────┐  ┌──────────────┐
│              │  │  Free Time   │
│              │  │    Kids      │
│              │  │   Family     │
│    Work      │  │   Social     │
│              │  │  Exercise    │
│              │  │  Household   │
│              │  │  Creative    │
│              │  │ Misc., etc.. │
└──────────────┘  └──────────────┘
```

I used to see it this way, too. One of my goal columns is called "Writing," and it's something I've been working on for many years. For decades, I tried to wing it with writing time. Because writing was "creative," I somehow felt that it didn't have to be scheduled into my calendar each week and that I would just do it when I "felt like doing it." In other words, I was trying to shove my writing time into my "free time" box, which already had a whole lot of other stuff inside of it.

The problem was, when I shoved everything else *outside of work* into the "free time" box, my free time didn't feel open or free. It felt cramped and chaotic, it felt like I was rushing around doing a lot of things, yet I never seemed to find enough time to focus on writing. When I did find a spare half hour in between rushing around, I couldn't focus for long enough to get any writing done, because I wasn't giving myself enough space to actually do it in. Has something like this ever happened to you before?

You can ask yourself: *Are there some goals I'm trying to shove into the free time box that I should create a different focus box for instead? One that allows me to have consistent space to concentrate on what I'm trying to do?*

After years of trying to just casually schedule my writing time and not writing anything as a result, I finally realized I had to create consistent focus space for writing each week or it simply wasn't going to happen. So, I decided that every Friday, I would block off a three-hour chunk on my calendar just for writing and see if it would make any difference at all. And somehow, miraculously, it worked! Making regular space for writing actually helped me write. In fact, over the last five years, I've been able to write five books in a row as a result!

Sounds simple and obvious enough, right? Creating regular space for things you want to do actually *helps* you do these things. It starts with making a tiny decision to make things that are important to you important in your weekly schedule, too.

Now, every Friday, I open up a document and I tell myself it's time to write. Sometimes a whole lot happens, sometimes only a little. Sometimes even writing one sentence feels really very challenging to do and I barely type anything at all. But because I've been doing it for so long now, my general expectation for Fridays is that there will be a wide range of writing experiences happening, and that I can't always predict which experience I will get.

However, I *can* predict that I will show up on Fridays. I will pull the "writing time box" out of the time wardrobe, I will put it on the table, and I will open it up. I won't open up four other boxes at the same time. I won't get distracted rummaging through other boxes on the shelves. I will take it one box at a time.

I will sit there for the same scheduled three-hour block each week and stare at a blank page in front of me, and just see what happens next. And then, usually, when I make this tiny, determined decision to simply plant myself there for that designated period of time, my brain will eventually decide to type something, since it can only hold onto its own irrational resistance and avoidance for so long. Because even though I love to write, my brain will almost always resist starting to write anything, it's just a strange little dance we do that I'm very familiar with by now.

Can you relate to this in some way? Does your brain sometimes try to resist and avoid doing things you actually like to do?

I've learned to remember it like this:

> *You've got to outlast your own brain's resistance with your own gentle determination and persistence.*

"*Gentle persistence*" means we treat it like an experiment, with far less criticism and judgement, and with much more curiosity about our own journey. You might say encouraging, gentle things like, *"Let's just see what happens if I sit here every week at the same time and try to do this thing,"* or *"Let's just take this one step at a time each week and see where it goes next,"* as though you are conducting a scientific experiment on your own brain.

Creating consistent space for things that matter can make all the difference for you. If you think about it, you already show up consistently in terms of time for your job. You already make space for work; you show up during the same hours. Some days, you do a small amount of work; other days, you do a whole lot. Still, you keep showing up for a familiar and consistent chunk of time each week. And, as a result, you move things forward regularly, because you're giving work consistent *space and time* in your schedule.

We can start to do this with other things that matter to us outside of work and get the same result by doing so. Start showing up more consistently for things you want to do, and you will start to move those things forward, one step at a time.

It's helpful to remember:

When we create space and show up consistently, what we're working on will naturally start to progress.

Small steps add up! You can take small steps to do really big things, you just need to create space where all those small steps can happen.

You can remember it like this:

- Create a *time box* for things you truly want to get done on a regular basis.

- When you pull out that *time box*, give yourself enough reasonable space and time in which to consistently do those tasks each week.

- Take it one box at a time, and one task at a time.

- Show up for yourself at the regular time you've set aside, and you'll naturally start to make progress with your chosen pursuits.

- Show kindness to yourself no matter what happens each week. Don't beat yourself up on the slow weeks; instead, tell yourself, *"Good job for showing up today."*

- Make a tiny decision to be determined in your gentle persistence and see what happens next!

The Time Boxes

What will you call your *time boxes*? We can start with the names of our three columns from our goals map, with "self-care" being one of them.

For example, my three goal columns include:

- Work
- Writing
- Self-Care

So, my *time boxes* would look like:

| Work | Writing | Self-Care |

What do yours look like? Write them out on paper inside of individual squares.

In addition to our goal boxes, let's consider adding in boxes that reflect our *core values* as well. *Core values* are things which are meaningful to you that you want to start to prioritize more consistently in your schedule.

For example, if "spending quality time with your kids and family" is important to you, create a *time box* called "Kids/Family." This "Kids/Family" box is something you will now prioritize instead of just trying to wing it each week. What do you want to do with your kids and family this week? How can you protect time for this purpose in your schedule a little more? Define this clearly for yourself so that you can set aside enough time to do it. And then, treat it as though it's nonnegotiable, and schedule it in your calendar accordingly.

Sometimes clients create a "Relationship" time box, where they are clearly defining what they want this to look like in terms of time together with their partner so that they can make space to do more things as a couple more regularly. Other clients have chosen "Friendship" as a core value, and some have chosen things like "Fun," "Learning," or "Community."

What *core values* do you want to make consistent time for in your schedule?

> *Ask yourself: What core values do I want to prioritize more right now?*

From now on, we're curating what goes into our time wardrobe and treating those select items with more kindness, attention, and care.

Organizing Your Boxes

Let's visualize putting all your time boxes, including both the ones for goals and for core values, back into the wardrobe closet and neatly arranging them on the shelves. Mine would look something like this:

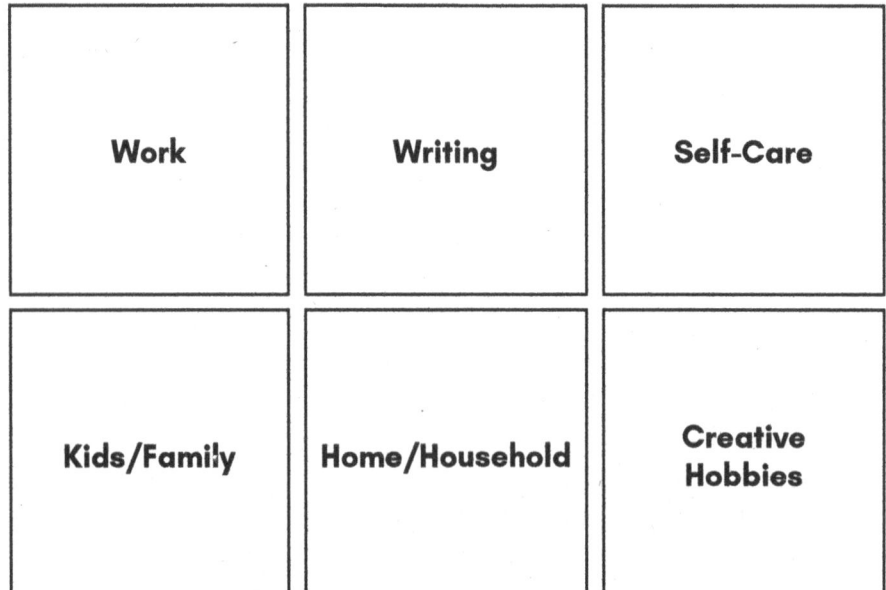

Remember, this closet is your weekly schedule. So, what do these *time boxes* look like on your actual weekly calendar? Let's try dropping them into our weekly schedule as *blocks of time*. First, we can look at each time box and then make a prediction for how much time it's going to require this week. Only how do we figure out what an accurate time estimate is for a task we need to do?

Realistic Time Estimates

When we're under a lot of stress, we may develop a kind of *time blindness* where we temporarily lose touch with our internal sense of time. In other words, our perception of passing time can become very wonky, and our ability to predict how long tasks will take us to complete starts to become really inaccurate as a result.

Have you ever thought something would take you ten minutes to do, but it actually took you two hours on the clock? Chances are you were under a lot of stress when you were making these types of inaccurate time predictions. And chronically making inaccurate time predictions tends to cause us to overbook our schedule on a regular basis. For example, if we think everything we need to do will take only a few minutes to complete, we will sign ourselves up to do many more things than if we think each of those tasks will take us a few hours to do.

If you find yourself going "time blind" on a chronic basis, it can be helpful to track how long tasks actually take you to do on paper, and then compare it to how long you thought they were going to take you in your imagination.

For example, you might track daily tasks like this:

Task	Time Estimate	In Real Time
Washing dishes	10 minutes	15 minutes
Answering emails	15 minutes	1 hour
Getting groceries	30 minutes	1.5 hours

Keeping track of your time estimates and comparing them to *real-time data* will help you realize where all your time is actually going, especially if you add up all the time you miscalculated for how long the tasks you needed to do really ended up taking. You can now allow yourself more than enough time to realistically complete tasks for the week.

Now, going back to our sample time boxes, let's take one time box and try to plan a realistic amount of time to do it in. For "Creative Projects," let's say we're working on a project that is going to require about four hours to complete that week. However, perhaps with everything else on our plate, finding one solid stretch of four hours is just too challenging for us to figure out right now.

We can now break this "Creative Project" box into two chunks of two hours on our calendar, and this makes it feel more manageable to find time in our schedule now.

Time	Monday	Tuesday
9:00	CREATIVE PROJECT	
10:00		
11:00		
12:00		
1:00		
2:00		CREATIVE PROJECT
3:00		
4:00		
5:00		

Break big things up into *small chunks that feel manageable to you*, and then find ways to drop these small chunks into *slots of time* where they feel easy for you to do, based upon your *predicted energy and stress levels* for that day.

To remember this:

- Prioritize your weekly goals and core values by sorting them into *time boxes.*

- Estimate how much time *each time box* will take you to do each week, and give yourself *much more than enough* time for tasks.

- For bigger tasks, break them down into tinier amounts that feel easier to manage.

- *Compartmentalize your time*: Take it *one box at a time* and *one task at a time.*

- Find slots of time in your calendar to drop your *time boxes* into that *match your energy and stress levels* for that day.

The Task Intensity Meter

So, how can we start to match our tasks to our energy levels each day? Here is an easy way we can start to look at which everyday tasks cost us the most energy to do, so that we can plan out our time more effectively each week.

Imagine a meter, with "low," "mid," and "high" written on it and a needle that swings between them all day long. I call this tool **"The Task Intensity Meter,"** and it's a tool I teach to everyone I work with. You can visualize it looking like this:

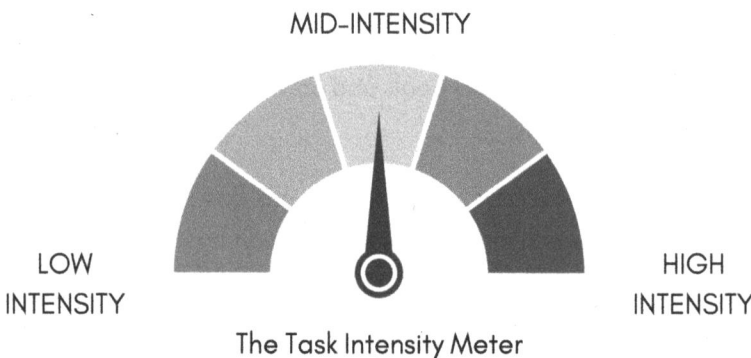

The Task Intensity Meter

When I say "intensity," what I mean is how stressful and intense this particular task feels for you to do. You would ask yourself, does the task I am doing feel *high, middle, or low intensity* to me right now?

Let's look at an everyday example so you can see how this works.

Task: Doing the laundry

Rating: Low/Mid/High?

How would you rate laundry right now for you as a task, would it be *low, middle,* or *high-level intensity*? You would be surprised at how often people tell me that laundry is a *high-intensity* task for them to do! I just want to normalize this so you can start to see that everyday tasks can stress people out far more than you might think. For many other people, while they don't love laundry, it also doesn't stress them out that much, so it's more of a *mid-level* intensity task for them. And there are some people who think doing laundry is not very stressful at all and others who even enjoy doing it, so they would rate it as a *low-intensity task*.

However, if doing laundry is a *high-intensity task* for you, what time of day would you choose to do laundry? Would you want to do it after you're already exhausted from working on other high-intensity tasks? Or would you now think about making it easier on yourself by doing it at another time instead? In this way, you can begin to match your scheduling of high-intensity tasks with times of day when you have the most energy to do them.

Try to write out a list of tasks you have to do today. Then, rate each task as low, middle, or high intensity, depending on how stressful it feels for you to do today.

For example, here is one client's list, a parent who works from home:

Task	Intensity Rating
Morning school run (dropping kids off)	Low
Laundry	High
Answering emails	High
Work meetings	Mid
Afternoon school run (picking kids up)	Low
Finishing work requests	Mid-High
Cooking dinner	High
Spending time with kids	Low
Reading a book before bed	Low

Looking at this list of task ratings, how might we schedule lower intensity tasks between some of the high-intensity tasks so the day isn't so stressful? We can ask ourselves something like, *"Can I avoid doing laundry right before starting work whenever possible? Can I save it for the weekend or a different time instead?"*

Play around with arranging your everyday tasks on paper, and see what solutions you can come up with to make things easier on yourself.

Ask yourself: How would I rate the tasks I have to do today? Write out your tasks and then rate them as low, middle, or high intensity. Then see how you can arrange them in an easier way.

Just by becoming more aware of which tasks tend to feel *high intensity* to you can really start to help you find ways to make things easier on yourself each week.

Here are some general guidelines to get you started:

Try not to stack too many high-intensity tasks in a row on top of each other. Each *high-intensity* task you do will cost you mental, emotional, and physical energy. Since most people tend to feel a certain level of stress after doing even one *high-intensity* task, give some thought to how doing two or three in a row might make you feel afterwards. Whenever possible, try to avoid stacking them back to back, and then make sure to give yourself enough space to reset after doing any *high-intensity* task so that you can bring your stress down a little.

Match high-intensity tasks with high-energy times of day. Plan the *highest intensity tasks* for when you have the *most energy* to tackle them. What times of day do you typically have the most energy? Some people find early mornings to be the best time to focus, but for some, it's afternoons, and for others, it's late at night. Pick the best times for you to do *high-intensity* tasks.

Whenever possible, give yourself *time buffer breaks* after high-intensity tasks. Leave some buffer space to bring the stress down after you've worn yourself out with a challenging task. Let yourself rest and reset before you launch right into doing something else. *Time buffer breaks* are about bringing your stress down in small degrees in between difficult things you need to do.

Everyone has a daily high-intensity task threshold. For some people, this might be one to two *high-intensity* tasks per day; for another person, maybe it's three or four per day. However, thinking you can accomplish dozens of highly stressful tasks in one day is probably a really unfair expectation to have of yourself on a regular basis. While you can push through and do something like this once in a while in a jam, you can't do this every single day without tipping yourself over into stress and burnout fairly quickly. Learn what your own threshold is, and try to avoid taking on too many challenging tasks in one day whenever possible. Try to space them out a little to make it easier on your brain and well-being.

Acknowledge and accept what's high intensity for you. Part of being kinder to yourself on a regular basis is acknowledging when things feel high intensity for you to do. Some days, certain tasks will feel *high intensity* to take on that weren't so challenging to tackle only a few days before. On other days, you will have so much energy that you will be able to tackle *high-intensity* tasks with greater ease. Our bodies, our stress levels, and our schedules all frequently go through changes, so we can show ourselves a little more compassion by adopting a nonjudgmental stance about what tasks are feeling hard for us to do right now.

Ask yourself: What everyday tasks feel high, middle, or low intensity for me to do?

Write out a few tasks and rate them (high/middle/ low intensity).

We can use the **Task Intensity Meter** for rating our own tasks, and we can have our kids rate the intensity of their homework and chores. Just like our **Stress Scale**, we can use the **Task Intensity Meter** as a communication tool to help our family understand how tasks emotionally affect us in different ways. Everyone's brain is different, and people are all over the place as to which tasks feel difficult for them to do each week.

You won't necessarily know what your family's *high-intensity* tasks are unless you ask them.

For example, using the **Task Intensity Meter** helped one of my kids decide which homework he should do first. When an assignment feels harder for him, it's easier for him to work on it right when he gets home from school, rather than delaying working on it until after dinner. However, this is not the case for my other kid; his energy usually improves after dinner, and it's much easier for him to do homework later at night. So, if I expected them both to do their homework right after school, this would only work effectively for one kid! However, I can use this tool with both of them and help them figure out when their own brains work best by writing it out together.

If you compare how my husband and I rate things like going to the store, he would probably rate it as slightly higher intensity for him than I would, and vice versa with other errands that I find much harder to do than he does. Perhaps we might discover that there are chores that are difficult for both of us, in which case, maybe we can alternate doing them, or divide them up more evenly so one person doesn't feel like they're doing all the *high-intensity* chores all the time.

We can gather information about which tasks stress people out and start to form some strategies in response by staying flexible and adaptable to the information we're receiving. Start by asking everyone to rate everyday tasks like laundry, cooking, going to the store, or doing the dishes, and see what you discover. This exercise can lead to fresh insights, new strategies, and much more empathy for each other, as well as more effective communication going forward.

Breaking Down Bigger Tasks

We can use the **Task Intensity Meter** as a way to break down big tasks into smaller pieces and see which pieces are making us feel stuck. Often, we're procrastinating on doing an entire task because of only one tiny piece of it that we find *high-intensity* to do. Once you realize what this challenging piece of the task is, you can change your approach and move out yourself out of procrastination in an easier way.

For example, let's take one client's example task: 'Planning a Trip.' Within this one task, there will be parts that will feel very easy, parts that will feel hard, parts of the task that will feel neutral. You can break the task down and give each piece of the task an intensity rating.

Task: Planning a Trip	Rating
Research flights	Low
Book flight	Mid
Book hotels	Mid
Pack suitcase	Low
Arrange activities and transportation	High

Looking at this breakdown, which piece requires the least energy to do and feels the easiest? Maybe researching flights would be an easy place for you to begin. After looking at this list, you might also want to save the activities and transportation part of this task for a time when you have the most energy to tackle it.

Let's consider another example from a client:

Task: Writing an Essay	Rating
Research paper	Mid
Write outline	High
Write pages	Mid
Edit pages	Low
Turn in paper	Low

For this particular person, they might now be able to predict that they will feel the most stuck when starting their outline. However, after making their list, they can see that once the outline's done, they will soon move on to the lower intensity parts of their paper, which will be much less stressful for them to do. So, they can plan to do the outline when they have the most energy to tackle it, and then remind themselves that the easier parts will soon follow.

By identifying the smaller parts of a big task that are making you feel stuck, you can start to help yourself develop workarounds for sticking points and roadblocks you might face.

Ask yourself: What parts of tasks do I tend to feel stuck on?

How can I help myself more with my approach to doing these stressful parts of the task?

Reward Yourself

If you find that you're getting stuck on a *high-intensity task*, try using rewards as a way to motivate yourself to complete it. Every time you finish a challenging task, plan a small reward for yourself afterwards. If rewards are something that you struggle with selecting, you can also save doing a *low-intensity* task that feels fun to you for after you've completed a harder task. For example, if grading papers for my class feels difficult for me to do, I can save something that feels easier for me to do, like buying tickets to an event I want to attend, as a *reward* for finishing doing grades. In this way, I can save the best task for last in order to motivate myself to do the hard task in front of me.

You can also play around with delayed gratification as a reward, too. Save watching that new episode of your favorite TV show as a reward for completing that *high-intensity* task you're stuck on. By putting off watching the episode until after you've completed the task, you can let yourself feel like you've earned it, and you'll probably enjoy watching the episode more having done so.

You can vary the rewards to match the size of the task; use smaller rewards for smaller tasks and bigger rewards for bigger tasks. Most importantly, save the most fun rewards for completing the tasks that feel the least fun for you to do.

Activating Your Energy

Typically, we want to feel motivated before we start doing a *high-intensity task*; however, most of the time, motivation tends to kick in after we've already started working on tasks. Motivation tends to strike moving objects, so if we're waiting for motivation to start moving us forward, we might be waiting for quite a while. Instead, we can ramp up our own energy to start moving first, and then find our motivation as we go.

Activation energy is a term used in chemistry to describe the minimum effort needed to get a chemical reaction. In psychology, we use *activation energy* to mean the minimum level of effort needed to move ourselves forward a little. We can ramp up our activation energy by establishing time parameters to do the task in.

Brain Boost:

When you have a set amount of time in which to do a task, your brain can help you do the task more effectively. Researchers from Tel Aviv University had participants take a test that included 2,400 tasks that were divided up into different blocks of time. One group was told how many tasks they would have to do and how much time they had to do each set of tasks, while the other group was given no information about the number of tasks or the time limit. The first group, which knew the task time limits, performed faster and more accurately than the group that had no information. (Katzir, Emanuel, and Liberman, 2020.)

So, how do we set specific task time parameters to activate our focus?

Task Sprints: If someone told you to run around the block indefinitely, you probably wouldn't want to do it at all. But if someone told you to run around the block for just ten minutes, you might think, *"Well, ten minutes doesn't sound so bad, I can probably get through it."*

It's the same with focusing on a task that feels difficult for you to do. Tell yourself, *"I only have to do this task for ten minutes,"* and see if your brain rises to meet this new challenge with newfound interest. You've now taken on a task your brain wants to avoid and made it sound like a game. After you've done your first *timed task sprint*, take a break and step away from working on the task for a bit. Then, when your energy has reset, do another round and see how many sprints it takes to get your motivation to kick in. Once you're feeling fully motivated, you probably won't need to do the timed sprints anymore.

If we are prone to experiencing *time blindness*, we may lose track of our own internal sense of passing time when we're working on challenging tasks. Sometimes, this can lead us to *hyperfocus*, an intense concentration state where we get excessively zoomed in on doing one task for too long without taking any breaks. While shifting into *hyperfocus* can sometimes help us cram and finish tasks before a deadline, doing it on a regular basis can easily tip us over into feelings of burnout. It's not sustainable as a default mode for completing tasks because it stresses out your brain and rapidly exhausts your body.

Doing *task sprints* can keep you from slipping too far into *hyperfocus*, because you will be pacing yourself in a steadier way by taking frequent breaks. You can play around with what length of *time limit* might work best for your own focus, while still maintaining your overall sense of balance and calm. You can also find focus-based groups online where people do timed task sprints together (see the resources section at the end of this book).

Music as Activation: We may instinctively use music to motivate us when we're working out at the gym, but how about when we're doing the dishes, working on a creative project, or just trying to get through those last work emails at the end of the day? Studies have shown that music can motivate us in powerful ways, so why don't we use it more often for getting through everyday tasks? When we use the same playlist for the same task long enough, we create a *behavioral association* for ourselves. Now, when we hear that particular piece of music, we've conditioned ourselves to want to work on the task!

Brain Boost:

In three different studies over the last decade, researchers discovered that listening to different types of music influenced peoples' motivational levels and emotional states. Listening to fast-paced music increased participants' motivation to work out on exercise bikes; and the faster the music, the faster people pedaled. In a different study, after listening to relaxing music, participants felt much calmer overall and performed better on a stress test. And in a third study, researchers found that listening to upbeat music while doing a task increased cognitive processing and improved memory skills for the participants. (Cherry, 2019.)

What energizing *task anthems* will inspire you to do those dishes or answer those emails this week?

Movement as Activation: When we're mentally stuck with tasks, we are often physically stagnant, too. We might be sitting down for long stretches of time, lost in our own anxious thoughts, ruminating about problems or future concerns. So sometimes, the best way to get that activation energy flowing is to move. Move your body a little, stretch your arms, or go for a short walk. Our bodies need to move around frequently; it helps our focus, it helps our attention, it helps our circulation, and it helps our sense of general well-being.

Often, all you may need to do to activate your focus is simply to move yourself to a new location. Go to a different room. Work at a different table. Can you take your task somewhere else to work on? Can you find another space that gets that activation energy flowing?

Mix things up when you're feeling stuck. Do something different for your brain! See if moving around physically starts to get your activation energy moving a little.

Inspiration & Intention: We can use *visual cues* to inspire us to take that first step forward. What *visual cues* might work for you? Inspiring quotes, pictures of places you want to go, or a photo of someone you admire? Put your inspiring *visual cues* where you can see them while you're working on your task. Use them to cue your brain to keep moving forward.

A client was trying to complete her PhD, but she was feeling burned out and unmotivated. She couldn't get herself to move forward with finishing the very last pages of her thesis. When I asked her what she was planning to do as a reward for completing the paper, she told me that she really wanted to spend a day at the beach. So, she decided to put a photo of a local beach above her computer as a *visual cue* to help her complete her thesis. After staring at the beach photo for a few weeks, she was finally able to finish writing the final pages. And after she finished, she drove herself to the beach pictured in the photo to celebrate.

"I got so used to looking at the photo of the beach and picturing myself there that when I finally arrived, it just felt really natural because I had already practiced it in my imagination," she later said in a session. "Because of doing that visualization, I could really let myself feel good about everything I had completed when I finally got to the beach."

That's how powerful visualizations can be to our brains: We can use them as maps of where we want to go, both physically and emotionally.

We can also use *setting intentions* as a way to activate our energy. Why do you want to do this task or goal? What do you want to feel afterward? Who will you help by completing this goal?

Write it out in a clear sentence on paper: *"I want to accomplish (fill in the blank) so I can feel (emotion) and so I can help (fill in the blank)."* For example, *"I want to finish this organization project so I can feel calmer and so I can help my family find things more easily."*

If you're not sure what to write, you could just say something about helping yourself by doing the task, such as, *"I want to complete this task so I can prove to myself I can do it, then I can feel relieved and enjoy my weekend."*

By stating your intention in a simple sentence, you're telling your brain that now there's a clear plan and purpose for your actions.

Our Energy & Expectations

It can be helpful to scan your current overall energy level on a regular basis by sitting still for a brief moment, closing your eyes, and asking yourself: *"How much general energy do I actually have right now?"* Then, try to really listen to what your body tells you for a few moments.

Do you have a lot of energy, a little bit of energy, or are you close to empty and running on fumes? Just as we don't always notice what our stress levels are, we often don't take accurate readings of our own energy levels either.

Doing this kind of *energy scan* helps us to get really honest about how much energy we actually have, instead of defaulting to thinking we "should have energy" to do all the things on our to-do list and then beating ourselves up about not being able to accomplish them all. For example, there are some days where I think "*I really should have a lot more energy*" because my schedule is fairly light, but when I do a quick energy scan, I realize I don't have energy at all, since I'm still recovering from a few stressful days in a row. I can then acknowledge where my energy level actually is and readjust my expectations accordingly. Although my schedule may be light on such a day, my energy is low, so maybe I'll select a lower-level intensity task to do instead of a higher one.

Sometimes where we're getting stuck with things is that we aren't adjusting our expectations to match our current energy levels in present circumstances. For example, are your kids home from school for the summer? Maybe it's time to lower our expectations a little about getting a lot of things done during this time window of their summer vacation from school. You'll probably be facing more interruptions and demands on your time, and it may be a lot harder to focus on things. Or are you home with the flu this week? Chances are you just won't have the energy to get things done to the same degree as you will when you're feeling better.

Slow down a little to take stock of your own energy, then make any needed adjustments to your own expectations about what you're able to do during this particular stretch of time.

You can get even more specific about noticing the different types of energy you have each day. Some days we have a lot of physical energy to do physical tasks, but we have completely run out of emotional energy to deal with any more problems. Other times, our physical and emotional energy levels are okay, but our neural energy feels depleted from focusing on a lot of difficult tasks in a row. Maybe it's time to get outside, take a walk, and shift into using our physical energy for the next segment of time. Or perhaps it's time to just take a break completely and let our brains fully reset instead. You'll be able to figure out what the next best step is for you as you become more consciously aware of what different types of energy feel like in your brain and body.

If you find that you still want to work on goals during periods of general low energy, you may want to stick with tackling lower intensity tasks during this time and save the middle and high-intensity tasks for when you feel more recharged and refreshed.

The more nuanced you can become about discovering all the different ways your various types of energy can fluctuate on any given day, the more you can take care of yourself and adjust what you're choosing to do with the next segment of time ahead.

> *Ask yourself: Thinking about the last few days, did I feel varying levels of physical, emotional or mental energy?*

Each day is a different story in terms of your energy levels. Things that felt easy yesterday may feel more challenging to do today, and vice versa. We have to take things one day at a time, one task at a time, one moment at a time, and adjust what we're trying to accomplish accordingly.

Go easier on yourself by being fair-minded and showing yourself some kindness and compassion. You're not a robot—you're allowed to change and fluctuate each day! It's all part of being wonderfully human.

Naming Your Days

Once you know what your *time boxes* are, you can try using a simple tool I call "**Day Labels**." It's a way to create a desired behavior association with a particular day of the week in order to really prep your brain ahead of time to do a specific task.

When I was in elementary school, the school cafeteria had "Taco Tuesdays," which caused quite a stir with the students. The tacos weren't particularly good, but the marketing was incredible. *"It's Tacoooooooo Tuesday!"* the school principal would announce cheerfully each Tuesday on the intercom. Flyers of dancing tacos lined the walls of the cafeteria with the words *"Taco Tuesday!"* in a happy bold font. Kids would say, *"Hey, guess what day it is? Taco Tuesday!"* to each other at recess, and by lunchtime, there would be a huge line out the doors of the cafeteria. The tacos always sold out. Everyone wanted a taco!

When you're a little kid, school days can often blend together into an endless blur of classes and assemblies, and something like "Taco Tuesday" marked something special happening in the week. In other words, Taco Tuesday became a special marker of time.

We need more special markers of time now as adults. We need to break up the monotony of our days with reminders about what we want to focus on today. When we give ourselves clear time markers to latch onto, our brains can help us more effectively plan out our schedule.

My **Day Labels** tool works like this: Make a "Taco Tuesday" for your brain to latch onto. For me, I might define each Friday as "Writing Friday," and if I call them this for enough weeks in a row, my brain will understand that's what's happening on Fridays now. For other clients I've worked with, they've named days "Walking Wednesday" for remembering to go on a long walk mid-week for self-care, or "Money Monday" for the day they add up all their business expenses in a spreadsheet each week. I even had one client use "Sunday Slowdown" to help her remember that on Sunday mornings, she needed to slow down for a few hours, put away her phone, and sit in her garden to be more present with the day.

This works well for goals we want to focus on, but you can also use it for household tasks and chores. By designating something like "Supermarket Saturday" in your weekly calendar, what you're really doing is minimizing the decisions you're going to have to make this week. Now, instead of just thinking, *"I'm going to the store whenever there's a free moment in my schedule,"* and then winging it, you're telling yourself, *"Saturday is the day I go to the supermarket."*

If you *name the day* consistently enough, your brain will now naturally scan your schedule each Saturday for an open time when you can go to the store. Then somehow, like magic, you'll find yourself doing that very thing on the particular day you named!

In this way, we're programming our minds for a task we want to do in the future by giving our brain something to latch onto and remember. "Taco Tuesday" worked because it felt happy, the principal made it seem entertaining, and the flyers of dancing tacos looked fun. If it had been a dreary announcement about tacos, along with unappetizing images of the actual tacos you were going to have to eat, nobody would ever have lined up for Taco Tuesdays. In other words, sell the task to your own brain by making it seem special, interesting, or different to do.

Decision fatigue happens to us all day long, and it's often spiking our stress levels way up high. The more tired we become, the harder decisions are to make and the more stress we will experience as a result.

Get yourself out of that weekly decision fatigue loop by telling your brain what exactly what it has to do on a particular day. Train your brain to get ready to take on whatever the task equivalent of "Taco Tuesday" is for you by naming your days and creating special markers of time.

The Hats Method

Here's another simple method to help you tell your brain where you want it to go and how to get there. It helps you prepare your brain for the task ahead so you can direct your focus and attention to what's next.

Imagine you're standing back in front of your time wardrobe. Only before you pull out a time box, you must select a corresponding imaginary "hat" to wear first. This represents the *mental gear* you must shift into as you open up this time box and work on the tasks inside.

We wear many imaginary "hats" throughout the week. For example, in the course of a week, I will wear a "writer hat," a "family hat," a "work hat," and a "teacher hat" because these are the different jobs, roles, and responsibilities I take on each week.

If I were to imagine these "hats" hanging on the wall on a rack, they might look something like this:

THE HATS METHOD

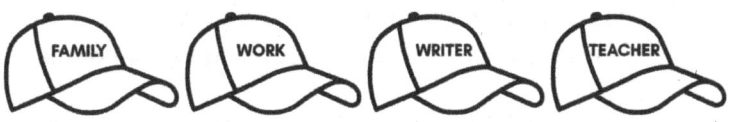

Ask yourself: What roles and jobs do I wear different "hats" for throughout the week?

Write them out on paper and label each one.

I call this "The Hats Method," and it's an easy visualization to help you learn how to narrow your focus down to what's directly in front of you. You can ask yourself, *"Which "hat" do I need to wear for the next upcoming segment of time?"*

Of course, I'm always the same person while wearing all my different "hats," and there are lots of overlaps in the skills I need to access when I'm wearing any of them. However, I feel like I'm using a different *mental gear* when I'm writing compared to when I'm doing therapy, and I'm in a different *mental gear* when I'm *teaching classes* as opposed to *helping out my own kids as a mom.*

Some hats, like my "family hat," are roles that I embody all the time, because I never stop being a mom to my kids or a wife to my husband. However, for me, thinking about taking off my "work hat" and putting on my "family hat" helps me to make an intentional shift back into the present moment to focus on my family and to put my work tasks aside. It reminds me that I'm there to connect with my kids and husband during this designated time frame, as opposed to checking my emails or doing dozens of other tasks I need to do. In other words, it helps me compartmentalize my focus and my time down to what's happening in front of me.

Using the "Hats Method" can help you:

Avoid multitasking. You'll learn that you can only wear one "hat" at a time if you really want to effectively direct your focus toward what's in front of you. With practice, you learn to put on the right hat for the corresponding time box. You learn to intentionally shift *mental gears* to where you need them to be.

Transition between things in a calmer way. After you practice this visualization tool for a few weeks in a row, you'll start to notice that you are learning to shift between different "hats" in a calmer way. Sometimes, you might do this by taking short *time buffer breaks* while you are transitioning between "hats." For instance, after taking off my "work hat," I will sometimes go for a quick walk around the block. As I'm walking, I think about what gear I need to shift into next and what "hat" I will put on when I return home again. This way, I've prepared my brain for the next segment of time ahead, and when I return, I'm often feeling much more motivated to tackle my next set of tasks.

Stay present in the moment. As you put on each new "hat," you are shifting back into the present moment again. You're reminding yourself what the next segment of time is for, and you're getting really intentional about where you will direct your focus next. You're pulling yourself out of your busy thoughts and into the "now."

Setting intentions. Each time we visualize putting on a new "hat," we are setting an intention for our next time segment of time. We can make this visualization work even more effectively for us if we actually state our intention in a simple sentence as we picture ourselves changing "hats." For example: *"For this next time segment, I'm going to focus on helping my kids with their homework,"* or *"For this next hour or two, I'm going to put on my "work hat" and get through all of my emails."* When you put on the "hat," tell yourself a statement of clear intention for what you intend to do with your time, and then your brain can help you get there.

See yourself with more compassion. When you begin to understand just how many "hats" you're wearing throughout your week, you'll start to have a whole lot more compassion for yourself. You can pull back and get a higher level perspective on everything you're doing, all the roles you play, and the various things you're responsible for. You'll start giving yourself a whole lot more credit for all of the diverse tasks you have to manage.

Wearing Too Many Hats

Often, we can get ourselves into trouble because we're trying to wear too many "hats" at once. Metaphorically, this means we are multitasking and jumping from one task to another without ever really focusing our attention directly on anything in front of us. Before we know it, we're completely mentally exhausted even though we haven't even finished anything we've set out to do!

In other words, we have burned through all our energy by wearing too many "hats" at the same time.

Have you ever had days like this? Do you ever think, *"What did I actually do today? How did I not manage to finish even one task completely, yet now it's night time?"*

One client described it like this: "All I do is run around all day long, and then it's dinner, and I haven't even finished even one thing! But I am so tired, it feels like I have done a thousand things. I just don't know where all of my energy and time goes."

To simplify this down, when we're caught in this pattern, we're just trying to pile too many hats on top of each other. Everything is taking up too much space in our minds as a result, and we're seeing it all as being at the same level of importance. You can picture it like this:

TOO MANY HATS

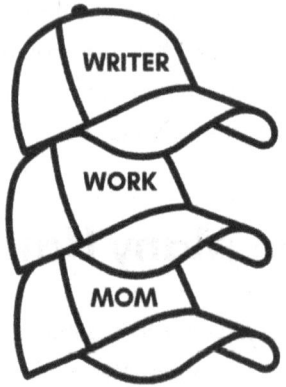

What does "wearing too many hats at once" look like in real life? If I put on my "family hat," "work hat," and "writer hat" all at once, I'm trying to help my kids with their homework, answer client emails, and write a paragraph of a book, all in the same hour, switching back and forth and never giving *anything or anyone* my complete focus and attention. And remember our stress scale? Chances are that my stress is climbing higher and higher on the scale as a result of all this task-jumping that I'm doing! And, emotionally, I'm probably getting grumpy with my kids, I'm getting frustrated writing a paragraph, and I'm forgetting important details in emails I'm sending to people.

Brain Boost:

According to Dr. Kevin Paul Madore at Stanford University, trying to multitask can create interference between the frontoparietal control network, the dorsal attention network, and the ventral attention network. This can often lead to slower processing time, forgetfulness, and making more mistakes while doing tasks, or as Dr. Madore calls it, "task switch costs," which results in a loss of accuracy or speed in doing a task. (*Neuroscience News*, 2021)

Wearing too many hats at once can stress us out, leave us fatigued, and cause us to make far more mistakes than when we slow down and just take it one task at a time. When we slow down and narrow our attention to what's right in front of us, we can figure things out much faster overall as well as finding our calm again.

Ask yourself: Which hats do I tend to pile on top of each other?

How does this tend to affect my moods and stress levels?

Take Off Your "Work Hat"

These days, many of us completely forget to take off our "work hats" for long stretches of time. We go to sleep with that "work hat" on, we wake up with it on, we go through the weekend with it on, and we go on vacations with our "work hat" stuck on our heads. Has this ever happened to you before? Have you ever spent the entire weekend thinking about work, only to feel mentally exhausted by Monday morning?

Why do we do this to ourselves? Why don't we let ourselves take off the "work hat" when work hours are over?

I really believe this is the reason so many people are feeling so very burned out these days. People just aren't taking their "work hats" off consistently and deliberately enough at the end of each day.

Brain Boost:

According to APA's Work and Well-being Survey of 1,501 adult workers in the US, 79 percent of employees had experienced work-related stress during the previous month before the survey. Nearly three in five employees reported negative impacts caused by work-related stress, including lack of interest, motivation, or energy (26 percent) and lack of effort at work (19 percent). 36 percent reported cognitive weariness, 32 percent reported emotional exhaustion, and 44 percent reported physical fatigue. (Abramson, A., 2022)

Take your "work hat" off each day, and make sure to give your brain a real break from thinking about your job. You can tell yourself, *"It's time to take off my "work hat" for today. I can think about all these things in the time I've scheduled for it tomorrow. But tonight, right now, it's time for me to relax and reset myself."*

You can give yourself permission to put that "hat" away when work is over. You can show yourself so much more kindness and compassion in this way.

Put the Hats Away

Ideally, we need more than a few occasions per week when we "hang up all of our hats." Maybe this is what you can redefine for yourself as your *calm zone*, perhaps as something you do regularly on your self-care goal column. Just like putting *time buffer breaks* in your calendar, give yourself some *mind buffer breaks* as well, where there is just free and open space to *be* without having to do anything at all.

We can tell ourselves these types of soothing phrases when it's time to "hang up our hats" for the day:

"I can allow myself to reset and relax right now. I don't need to do anything or be anything right now."

"Tomorrow I can figure out what I need to do, one step at a time. I don't need to think about anything else tonight."

"I can let my brain have a break right now. It's worked really hard all day, and I can allow it to rest."

"I did enough for one day. I can let things go for a little while. Everything will be waiting for me tomorrow."

Tomorrow, you can pick up a "hat" to wear again. But tonight, you can let yourself fully reset first.

The Morning Reset

Mornings can be an especially stressful time, some of which can be blamed on our bodies' *cortisol awakening response*, which tends to shoot our stress hormones way up just as we awaken into consciousness. And then, in this stressed-out state, it's easy for a wave of unhelpful mind chatter to hit us before we've even moved our bodies out of bed.

"I have so much to do! I'll never get it all done! How will I do everything ahead of me?" we might think before we've had a chance to put our feet on the floor.

Brain Boost:

Our cortisol awakening response may come from primitive times, according to Dr. Carlos Contreras: "The diurnal secretion of cortisol occurs near the time of awakening (i.e., after a period of rest or sleeping) and persists for several hours in the absence of any current stressful situation. The CAR (cortisol awakening response) seems to represent an ancient adaptive-allostatic feature that prepares an individual to face eventualities that are forthcoming during the day." (Contreras and Gutiérrez-Garcia, 2018, p.29.)

To counter this primitive reaction, we can practice something I call "**The Morning Reset**" and find ways to center ourselves in calm at the start of each day.

Each morning is a chance for you to reset and start again. We don't have to carry yesterday's moods into today. We can start each new day with a clean slate.

To use this tool, you just have to do two simple things.

The Morning Reset

- When you wake up, tell yourself one encouraging thing.

- Then slowly get up and do one thing to gently ease yourself into the day.

Here are some examples of encouraging things you can tell yourself when you first wake up:

- *"Every day I can start over. Each morning I can reset myself and begin again."*

- *"There are so many possibilities for this new day. I can stay open to new possibilities."*

- *"I don't have to bring yesterday's moods into today. I can start with a clean slate."*

- *"Every day is a day I haven't seen before."*

- *"Each new day is one I have never experienced. I am going to embrace this new experience."*

- *"New things can happen today, and I'm going to try to notice them more when they do."*

- *"I'm going to show myself kindness by just taking it one step at a time."*

- *"I can go at my own pace. I don't have to rush. I can slow down on purpose."*

- *"Each new day is a chance to learn and grow."*

Find an encouraging phrase that resonates with you to tell yourself when you're just waking up, then say it to yourself each morning consistently for a few months in a row and see how it affects your mood as you go throughout your day.

The way you start out your day is important; it paves the emotional pathway for your brain and changes how you perceive things that will follow.

Brain Boost:

Researchers from the University of Pennsylvania studied how employees started their mornings and how it affected the rest of their day. Employees who started off the morning from a positive mindset had improved performance during the day, and they generally viewed their entire day from a more positive perspective overall. When employees started the day from a negative mindset, Wilk reported, "Employees could get into these negative spirals where they started the day in a bad mood and just got worse over the course of the day." (Rothbard and Wilk, 2011.)

Now that you've encouraged yourself with a morning affirmation, you can start to get out of bed and find a very gentle transition to ease your body into movement.

For some people, this gentle transition might be one of the following:

- Stretch for a few minutes. Let yourself slow down and feel what your body is feeling for a minute or two.

- Slowly walk around for a few steps, or slowly drink some water. Connect with your body as you're doing this, while giving your body and brain some time to align with each other.

- Write in a journal for a few minutes just to let your brain wake up gently and organize your thoughts for what's ahead.

- Take a few long deep breaths in and out before you get up and do anything.

Play around with whichever "gentle transition" works best for you to do consistently. You can remember the **Morning Reset** like this:

Say something kind to your brain and do something kind for your body each morning.

Have you ever shot out of bed and dashed around in a stress-induced frenzy before your tired brain even had a chance to come into consciousness? I know that for me as a parent, this happens quite a lot! I often throw myself right into making breakfast, getting kids up, brushing teeth, and packing lunches before my brain is even able to process what I'm doing. My body is moving on autopilot while my brain is still half-asleep, and what tends to happen? I'm spiking my cortisol levels way up before my brain even has a fair chance to take it all in.

These days, I make a point to slow down on purpose in the morning. When I want to speed up, I go even slower. When I feel myself rushing around, I sit down for a few minutes, take a few deep breaths, and remind myself, *"One day at a time, one step at a time, one moment at a time."*

We can learn to gently transition into our day with a little more kindness toward our brains and bodies from now on. We can slow down on purpose and make our way into the new day one step at a time. We don't have to frantically rush into the day or jump to conclusions about what the new day will be like for us.

You can allow yourself to be a beginner at today. After all, you have never lived through this particular day before! Be open to the day, ease into it a little more gently, slow down a little more.

After all, we all want more time, so why do we race through so much of the time we actually have? When you slow down with intention, you can find your flow again.

Chapter Four

Show Yourself Proof: Small Steps Add Up to Big Things

Acknowledge Your Progress

Do you remember a time when you wanted to be where you are right now? Do you remember a moment in the past when you wanted all the stuff you have right now? Do you remember years ago imagining doing some of the things that you're doing right now? Maybe it was driving a car, visiting new places, living in your own space, having a job, or getting to do fun stuff. Maybe a past version of you would look at Today You and think, *"Look how amazing that is, we get to do all that and have those things and go there and do that?"*

We so quickly tend to forget how things were *before*, and fail to remember all those tiny steps we had to take to get where we are *now*. However, we can learn to appreciate our own journey a little more by becoming an active and engaged witness to our own progress from now on. It's a simple way to start to befriend yourself, to cheer yourself on, and to learn to give yourself credit for everything you're doing and be mindful of it more of the time.

But how do we get our brains to more frequently acknowledge the small steps we're taking?

It starts with *showing your brain proof of your own progress as irrefutable evidence*. We can do this by tracking our tiny steps on paper in order to get our brain really on board with witnessing everything we're doing and how we're walking ourselves to places we want to go.

All of those "hats" you've been wearing, all of those tiny goal steps you're taking, and all of those time boxes you're organizing—it all counts, and we're going to show our brains that these things matter to us from now on.

Our Fickle Brains

Often, when I ask clients how they accomplished a big goal, these things tend to happen:

- They can't remember many of the small steps they took to get there.

- They can't remember how long each small step took them to do; also, depending on the goal, they sometimes can't even remember how long the entire journey took to complete.

- They can't remember the emotional place they were in *before* they took the first step compared to *after* they achieved their goal.

- If they aren't really feeling happy emotions about accomplishing their big goal, it's often because they are dismissing and ignoring all the actual work they put in to get there.

Why is it so important to remember all these things? The reason is this: If you remember how you felt before the journey started as opposed to where you are now, you can actually give yourself permission to feel proud of your own progress. In other words:

By acknowledging all of the steps you took along the way, you can really allow yourself to feel proud of what you've accomplished.

But why is it so hard for so many of us to really acknowledge our own progress? Why do we seem to forget so much of what we've done once we've accomplished what we set out to do?

Charles Darwin, who tracked everything he did every day in a journal, seemed to understand our brain's natural ability to forget things when he wrote, "Trust nothing to the memory; for the memory becomes a fickle guardian when one interesting object is succeeded by another still more interesting." (Chancellor, G., et al, 2009.)

Our brains truly are fickle guardians of the "truth." We get distracted, we forget things, we don't notice big events that happen, and we get much too zoomed in on absurd details that don't matter in the grand scheme of things. We brush over truly amazing things we do, and then we get stuck thinking about the one tiny thing we think we did wrong (sometimes for decades afterwards).

And we do this...a whole lot of the time!

For example, when I ask someone what they did over the last year, they will often only be able to tell me three to five things that happened. But hundreds, even thousands of things happened to them over the course of the year. So, which of these things do our brains choose to remember as keepsakes of the year?

For most of us, it's often a jumbled mess of small and big things, strange and negative things, fun emotions and not-so-fun ones. It's a vague, blurry, unsorted blob of stuff. People will say things like, "Let's see. Last year, I won an award. But then my car got in a fender bender, and I'm still sorting out the insurance. My kid graduated high school, but then I threw my back out and had to go to physical therapy for a month. If I think about it, I didn't do much of anything this year. It wasn't that great of a year!"

We are often so quick to dismiss the entire span of a year—*twelve months of time*—with only a few random snapshots of what took place over *a few hours* of time. But our year was comprised of incredibly many more snapshots than that! And some of the snapshots that we've lost along the way are the ones we would have instead wanted to store for posterity.

Unfortunately, our brains are still wired from early primitive times with a *neural negativity bias* that causes them to flag all of the dangerous and negative encounters as the most important ones to remember. We will almost always flag and store negative things that happen to us over things that may emotionally benefit us more to remember. Back in the cave days, this helped us survive imminent dangers such as bears and tigers attacking us in the wilderness. However, now that we're no longer being hunted down by wild beasts on a regular basis, this negativity bias just tends to stress us out unnecessarily.

Now, when you get an unpleasant work email from your boss, your brain flags it as really important to remember—never mind that it isn't an oncoming bear! However, it might feel like an oncoming bear to our nervous systems, and we will react accordingly in a really dramatic and stressed-out way. Did you just get a parking ticket? Our brains will flag this as the most important memory of the entire week! Never mind that a dozen pleasant things happened to you before you got that parking ticket. They've now all been replaced by the memory of that one silly parking ticket due to something called *negative memory bias*.

And when we talk about our goals, we tend to hold onto all of the frustrating roadblocks we faced along the way more than we hold onto the little triumphs of getting through those very same challenges.

Brain Boost:

Dr. Kenneth Yeager of the Stress, Trauma, and Resilience (STAR) Program at the Ohio State University's Wexner Medical Center claims there is a way to counter our negative memory bias: "The single most important underlying factor is how we talk to ourselves about our experiences. If you challenge yourself...to be mindful of your daily activities, noticing what's important [and what isn't], you are more likely to have positive life experiences," Dr. Yeager explains. By zooming in and getting your brain to notice the positive progress you're making more intentionally, you will have a better chance of remembering and storing these memories in the future.

This is why our brains need some sort of visual progress map to be able to see our journey toward our goals over a long stretch of time instead of relying solely on our own memory's sporadic and often fickle emotional snapshots of time. We need to show our brain proof of our progress so that we can connect with it emotionally and celebrate it more often.

The Small Steps Journal

Tracking our small steps in a nightly journal helps us to see our growth and our journey from a distance. I call this the "**Small Steps Journal**," and it helps you to witness and acknowledge your own progress over time so you can begin to cheer yourself on for all of those tiny goal steps you're taking each week.

And since we've already established our habit of writing out our **Magic Post-it** and our **Goals Map**, it's going to be very easy to do since we're just writing down the small steps we've already been taking in our **Small Steps Journal.**

Purchase a tiny notebook that you like. The style is entirely up to you. It shouldn't be that big at all; in fact, it's much better if it's smaller in size. It's not a diary where we're going to be writing pages and pages of details each day. Like many of my other tools in this book, it's going to be short and sweet and simple.

Every night, you're just going to write down any weekly steps you took toward your goal, however small they were, in a simple bullet list in this tiny bullet journal.

For example, one client's *three goal columns* were the following:

- **Column One: Creative—Painting**

- **Column Two: Work—Finish report by deadline**

- **Column Three: Self-Care—Weekly walking and/ or meditating**

Each day of the week, the client would write the steps they took on each of these columns in a bullet list in their **Small Steps Journal**, like this:

Monday

- Put paintbrushes out

- Wrote first few sentences of work report

- Meditated for five minutes

Tuesday

- Bought blank canvas online

- Wrote another piece of work report

- Went for a walk around the block after dinner

Wednesday

- Sketched out ideas on paper

- Finished a paragraph of work report

- Listened to a relaxing podcast

Thursday

- Sketched out more ideas

- Finished a draft of work report

- Walked one mile after dinner today!

Friday

- Organized paints and ordered some new colors

- Turned in work report by deadline!

- Walked one mile again!

In this example, you can already see how this client is moving themselves forward with things they want to do, in small daily steps. We can see how in only a few days' time, they were able to increase their short daily walk to one mile, and they were also able to finish a work report that was due by the deadline. And we can also see that they're starting to move forward with their painting, one tiny step at a time.

Not all your goal columns will move at the same speed. Some will take much longer to move forward, while others will move along very quickly. Some months, everything will be super speedy, while during other months, everything will grind to a halt. All of this is okay. We're just collecting data over time. We're not judging any of it. We're watching it, as interested and curious observers of our own time.

No step is too small to write down. If all you did was look something up online, write it down. Did you send an email to someone? Write it down. Did you manage to open a Word document and stare at it? Put it down! It all counts, from now on.

*Adopt a nonjudgmental stance toward
your own progress.*

*Witness each small step you take with curiosity
instead of criticism:*

"Where will this lead me next?"

Remember, the point of this **Small Steps Journal** is to collect data over a long stretch of time so we can show our brain our own progress on a visual map of our journey. See it as a scientific experiment to see how progress is unfolding in your life. Be open-minded; don't judge what you're putting in there, instead look at what you're doing through the eyes of curiosity: *Any small step counts. It all matters. It all adds up*!

In a way, through tracking your own progress, you learn to become a friend to yourself. You become your own witness, along for the ride and for all the ups and downs, and you'll start to encourage yourself throughout all of it. *"Keep going,"* is what you're saying simply by keeping this journal, *"Keep going, let's see what happens, let's see where all this leads us."*

From this stretched out space, we can begin to look at our journey as an interested observer, watching our own progress week to week, month to month, year to year. Where will this journey take us? Where will that little step lead? We really want to find out now!

Dancing with Time

When I was about five years old, my mother gave me an animation flipbook of a dancing mouse. It was a tiny little book only a few inches wide, and when you flipped the corners really fast with your thumb, it looked like a mouse was dancing a little waltz. It completely blew my five-year-old mind because it seemed like magic that the mouse could suddenly glide across the pages.

This is what your **Small Steps Journal** will be like for you. You will write down the small steps you are taking toward goals each day, and you won't really notice that much changing on a daily level. However, when you later flip through your little book at the end of the year, you're going to witness yourself moving forward by leaps and bounds. You'll see that the email you sent off in March finally paid off by May. That raise you requested in June finally arrived in December. The short story you started in July turned into significant chapters of the book you're writing by the end of the year.

It will have the "flipbook effect" for you in this way: It will seem magical how some things worked out in ways you could never have predicted, while other things seemed to follow a slower and steadier tempo the whole way through. In the end, it will help you connect the dots between all the small steps you have taken throughout the year, providing a more complete perspective on your overall journey.

Default to Appreciation

Some days, you might have a whole lot of things to add to your bullet list; other days you might only have a little. Some days, there might not be anything going on at all. Even when I only have one little bullet item to put down, I try to write three things down on the page anyway. On an occasion like that, I will add in things like rewards, treats, or even just happy moments from the day that I want my future self to remember.

Sometimes, when you don't have much to write down about your goal progress, it can be helpful to just default to appreciation instead. What did you appreciate from your day? Imagine Future You flipping back to this list later; what would Future You delight in reading about from today?

For example, going back to the client's list, let's say that on Friday, she didn't move forward with two of her goals because she had to focus all of her attention on finishing her work report. In this case, her **Small Steps Journal** entries might look like this:

Friday:

- Turned in work report by deadline!

- Had a really fun conversation with my sister and we started planning our next road trip

- Reward: Took myself out to the movies for finishing work report

Put down any treats, rewards, or delightful things from your day. Even if all you did was eat a nice salad or play with your pet dog, write it down. It will give you a little chuckle when you read that entry at the end of the year, and that's the point of this little journal. We want to delight in reading it later so when we look back on our time, we have given ourselves something to smile about.

Celebrate Your Successes

Some of my more artistically inclined clients like to draw celebratory drawings when they accomplish big wins in their

Small Steps Journal, and other clients like to use highlighters or stickers to mark when happy things happen throughout the year.

Mark up your notebook in whatever way feels fun or playful to you. That way, when you're flipping back through the pages, those items will visually stand out as special moments to remember. Circle those wins and happy moments, underline them, draw some arrows pointing to them, whatever you want to do! Connect with your successes when they happen, right there on the page in your own mini-journal celebration.

Compartmentalize Your Journals

If you start to feel frustrated or restless on certain days, or you feel any other intense emotions like fear, worry, or self-doubt, try to avoid writing these things down in this particular small journal. Save writing about more intense feelings you're experiencing or problems you're stuck on for a different notebook. Freewriting journals, where you let yourself pour out your feelings on paper without stopping yourself, can be a great to do this, but we want to keep this particular **Small Steps Journal** separate, so that it only reflects our weekly goal steps.

In the same way that we're learning to more effectively *compartmentalize our time*, we're now learning how to *compartmentalize our journals*, too. Trust me on this one, as someone who has kept all sorts of jumbled up journals at different stages of life, with pages full of frustrations, complaints, and long-winded passages about problems I didn't always want to read about later on. While these types of things are helpful to get off our chests in a notebook, what happens is it can become very hard on our future self's brain to sort out the enjoyable memories from the unpleasant ones when everything is mixed up together in this way.

Compartmentalizing this particular **Small Steps Journal** will make it special to you, and keeping this journal short and sweet will also encourage you to write in it more consistently.

"I only have to write three things down," you'll start to think, *"That only takes a few seconds to do, I can do that easily."*

Over time, if you write in the **Small Steps Journal** frequently enough, it might even become a nightly habit that you start to approach with a feeling of anticipation.

"I look for things now to write in my journal," one client said after keeping the **Small Steps Journal** for six months. "Now, if I complete something during the day, I think, 'I'm going to write this down later.' It's like I'm looking for the small wins on purpose, and collecting them feels more fun for me to do. And sometimes, I just write stuff down that makes me smile or laugh. I feel like I'm becoming my own friend just from writing in it each day."

Whatever you write in the **Small Steps Journal** will become a special keepsake of your entire year. In other words, make sure that from now on you're curating the things you actually want to hold onto in your memory banks.

The Yearly Review

At the end of the year, it's time to celebrate finishing your **Small Steps Journal** by reflecting upon all the progress you've made over the last twelve months. It's time to acknowledge your growth, progress, and learning by reading through all the pages and taking it all in.

So, set aside a half hour at some point in December to do a yearly flip-through of your **Small Steps Journal**. It's the most important and rewarding part of this goal-tracking experience, and it will help you feel really proud about everything you've done so far. It provides that *irrefutable evidence* that your brain needs to connect you with the feeling of completion that you've been really craving.

You will now feel "happy and done" when you read through all of your small steps across twelve months' worth of time. It just starts to happen naturally, just by flipping through it all and showing yourself proof of what you've done.

Sit somewhere relaxing and start to read through your pages. You'll see all the paths you took, the big things that happened, the slow times, the busy times, and all of those consistent small steps you took the whole year long. Savor it all a little. Revel in your own journey a bit. Enjoy your magical dance with time across the pages!

Then, on the very last blank page of the journal, write down a **Yearly Round-Up List** of anything you feel proud of from the year to close out the book. Put down at least one thing from every month of the year that makes you feel proud, delighted, or happy. Think of it as a spectacular *bullet list finale* to close out your **Small Steps Journal** and create a record of all the enjoyable and happy stuff you really want to remember for a long time afterwards.

When you close out the book, you're closing out the year.

You're saying thank you to the year. You're saying thank you for all the insights you gained. You're saying thank you for all the challenges that helped you grow. You're saying thank you for all the delights and joys you experienced. But mostly, you're saying thank you to yourself for everything you've done and learned this year.

Then, after you've reflected on the year, put away the journal. Keep it somewhere special and safe. Read it again from time to time whenever you need a little boost of motivation to remind yourself that you figured things out before, and you'll figure things out in the future, too.

Chapter Five

Embrace Being Done: Practice the Feelings You Want to Feel

The Phases of Progress

After tracking your small steps from a higher level perspective across enough time, you may now start to recognize your own *phases of progress* before they even happen.

In other words, with every goal or project you take on, there's going to be some sort of journey you embark upon. Just like the hero of an adventure movie, your journey will usually start with some sort of hesitation and doubt, but at some point, you will overcome both of these and take that very brave first step forward into the unknown. Then, you'll travel for a little while in small steps, learning new things and figuring things out until you inevitably hit a few roadblocks and obstacles along the path.

At this point, you will probably bump into your own insecurities and fears, and your confidence may even become very shaky for a moment. However, you will soon recover, and then, emboldened with a new sense of courage and determination, you'll complete your goal, one step at a time, and make it all the way to the end. When you finally cross your goal's finish line, you'll have become a stronger person from the entire journey, with all of its highs and lows. You'll have grown a lot, learned a lot, and you will now feel a whole lot more confident than when you started. You'll have acquired new knowledge to share with others and you'll have gained new skills from all the challenges you've overcome.

And then, you'll decide to take on the next journey and do it all over again! Some things will be the same, and some things will change. But over time, you'll start to see that there are some patterns you can now predict.

When you track your goals journey over enough years, you start to become more and more familiar with these types of patterns. In a way, this leads you to a whole new level of *self-kindness*, because now you'll be able to lighten up on yourself when you hit those inevitable bumps in the road. You can start to say things like, "*Yep—this happened last time. And somehow, I got through it, and I'm sure I'll do it again with this one.*" Or, "*I always seem to lose my confidence about halfway through projects no matter how many times I do this, but I know I will eventually tap into my inner strength again as I have done many times before to get past this particular stage.*"

Now, you've really become the "table sweeping mentor" that we discussed at the beginning of the book, and you'll also have become the *hero* of the journey, too. Your *inner mentor* can now actively encourage you from a higher level perspective as you navigate the terrain below.

"*Keep going!*" your inner mentor will say to you as you move down the path, "*That obstacle doesn't really look so bad, keep moving and you'll find a way around it.*" Or, "*Take a break and reset, we can do some more tomorrow from a clearer headspace."* Or, *"You're almost there, you've got this now!"*

This is how all of the various pieces of the *self-kindness mindset* start to really come together. You've taught yourself to break things down into tiny steps, you've taught yourself to regulate your internal dashboard of emotions and energy, and now, you are teaching yourself how to encourage yourself each tiny step of the way. And somewhere along the journey, you will have finally learned to *befriend yourself* and to really cheer yourself on, too.

When you reach this new level of *self-kindness*, then the feeling of completion and being done will really start to kick in for you with every small step you complete. You can now tell yourself things like, *"Great job, you did it, you finished another step! You're really doing this now! You've got this!"*

Then, after that point, comes the very last test of our journey—connecting with the praise and encouragement we're telling ourselves. Now that you're encouraging yourself more of the time, are you really hearing it and feeling it internally?

Ask yourself these questions:

- *Can I like myself during all the different phases of progress?*

- *Can I like myself when things are going slow?*

- *Can I like myself when I'm resting or taking a break?*

- *Can I allow myself to go at my own pace?*

- *Can I encourage myself more when I hit a roadblock or obstacle?*

- *Can I cheer myself on as I learn new things?*

- *Can I allow myself to be kind to myself consistently from now on?*

Expand Your Idea of Success

We can now come full circle back to the beginning of the book and compare our vision of success through the lens of a *toxic productivity mindset* vs. a *self-kindness mindset* by making two lists about what "success" means under each perspective.

What would go under each column for you?

Here's an example from a client:

Topic: What Success Means

Toxic Productivity Mindset	Self-Kindness Mindset
How much output I generate in a day	How I feel at the end of the day
How much money I make	How much well-being I let myself feel
How my success compares to others	How proud I feel about the things I do
How many milestones I reach	How kind and encouraging I can be to myself no matter what I'm doing
How fast I can achieve goals	Going at a pace that feels healthy to me
Doing everything perfectly	Embracing life-long learning, and knowing that I'm learning new things no matter what
How my life looks matters	How my life feels matters
I have to do and accumulate a certain amount to be successful	Figuring out the things that give my life meaning makes me successful

When we change what success means to encompass being kind to ourselves, it changes how we feel about what we do and allows us to emotionally connect with our feelings of completion.

For example, did you learn something today? Then you can let yourself feel done. Did you show yourself a little bit of kindness and encouragement today? Then let yourself feel done. Did you pace yourself in a way that allowed you to keep your balance? Then you did it! You're done!

Conversely, the other way, where we beat ourselves up to work faster and harder all the time in an attempt to do everything "perfectly," *never* allows us to feel done. We will never be able to do things fast enough or flawlessly enough, so there is never going to be a completion point for us to connect with emotionally. Think about this for a second, and you'll start to see how this could be a no-win situation you might be getting stuck in on a regular basis.

Instead, choose the path that lets you feel satisfaction with what you've done, as well as feeling calmer, rested and balanced, and happier more of the time!

Be Kind to Your Mind

The idea that we have to be "perfect" and achieve a certain "perfect" number of milestones in a "perfectly" limited amount of time may run so deep that we might not even know just how much intense pressure we are putting on ourselves each day. This internal pressure is also causing us to feel a lot of stress, which is probably *not* helping us get stuff done at all.

You don't have to put so much pressure on yourself all of the time. You don't have to create this extra stress for yourself to navigate every day.

The problem with perfectionism is that our "hustle culture" tends to actively encourage it, and people wear it like a badge of honor because they think it means they "won't settle for anything less than the best." Unfortunately, perfectionism doesn't help us achieve "the best" at all; more often, it just makes us feel more stagnant and stuck, which makes us feel like "the worst" as a result.

In reality, what perfectionism really means is that you've established *different rules for yourself* than you have for other people, and that these rules are impossibly unfair ones that you wouldn't have for anyone else but *you*. It's a way of being extra harsh toward yourself under the guise of "having high standards" that no human can actually meet.

Here's an example of how clients formed different rules for themselves as opposed to others in the exact same situations:

Situation: It took me over a year to complete my goal.

What I tell myself:	What I would tell another person:
"I would have been done so much faster, but I am lazy and took too many breaks. I am so far behind everyone else now!"	*"A year isn't that long at all to accomplish a really big goal. You should be so proud of yourself! You kept going, and look at what you've accomplished— that's amazing!"*

Situation: It took so long for me to start working on my goal.

What I tell myself:	What I would tell another person:
"I should have figured this out years ago, and I wasted so much time not moving forward. I should be much better at this by now! I'm such a mess."	"It often takes people a while to get started and to figure things out. And look how much progress you've made since you started. Keep going, you're doing great!"

Situation: I am really tired and have a headache, but I am so close to finishing this task.

What I tell myself:	What I would tell another person:
"I should just stop complaining and finish it now. If I just push through it, I can finish this if I stay up really late."	"Listen to your body. Take a break. You're going to feel so much better when you step away from this for a minute and reset yourself. Resting will help you feel better."

Reading these two columns, can you start to see how differently we tend to talk to ourselves compared to other people? Why wouldn't we talk to ourselves in the same way as we talk to others? Why wouldn't we treat ourselves with the same kindness that we treat other people with?

You are worthy of your own kindness and encouragement.

The words you say to yourself *matter*. Your brain is always listening to the words you're telling it. Be gentle and kind more of the time in the words you're telling yourself, and see how this starts to change the way you start to feel overall. Talk to yourself as if you are your own encouraging mentor from now on.

> *Ask yourself: "What would it feel like if I stopped being so hard on myself for a while? What would I do with all the mental space and energy that I now have available?"*

On a purely practical level, being chronically hard on yourself is burning through a lot of your energy each day, and it's also stirring up a lot of extra internal stress for you to experience. And while we can't control all the external stress coming at us each day, from now on, we *can* control some of the internal stress we are generating for ourselves.

Show yourself more kindness, encouragement, and love in small amounts each day. Give yourself enough time and space to learn, to grow, to experiment, to play, to focus, to have fun, to rest, and to learn new things, one step at a time.

Tell yourself you're proud of yourself, tell yourself you can do it, tell yourself to keep on going! Expand your definition of success so that you can see that you're constantly achieving it just by learning and growing each day.

In other words, every day that you learn something new or move forward a tiny step, you did it! You can count the day as a success.

Be consistently kind to yourself in this way.

And from now on, let yourself really feel happy and done with every single day.

Show Yourself Some Love

As we've made our way through the book, hopefully you're now starting to realize that this book isn't *just* about managing your time, staying balanced, and achieving your goals; it's really about learning to love and accept yourself, no matter what you happen to be doing! And that's really what all of it is about, isn't it? Achieving goals is just a way we learn to love and accept ourselves, and we can do that whether or not we're working on goals.

Accepting ourselves means learning to be honest with ourselves about how much energy we have and how much stress we're feeling on any given day. We can listen to what our brains and bodies are telling us more, and we can go at a pace that allows us to maintain our general happiness and well-being. We can create regular space to do the things that matter to us, and we can practice the feelings we really want to feel in daily amounts. We can allow ourselves to change and fluctuate as part of being human and make any ongoing adjustments along the way as needed.

We can figure things out, one tiny step at a time.

We can see ourselves as the hero of our own journey, and we can become our own mentor. Where will this tiny step lead us next? Where will this path take us? We really want to know now!

Because we realize that whatever path we're traveling down, we're always learning and growing. And that's the real adventure.

We can be kind to ourselves as we learn and grow, and we can encourage ourselves more of the time. And no matter what we decide to do next, we can accept and appreciate that we have intrinsic worth just by being alive.

So, if all you learned throughout the course of this book was to be a little kinder to yourself, then that's more than enough. Just by being kinder to yourself on a regular and consistent basis, you will start to change your whole relationship with your time, your goals, and more importantly, with *yourself*.

Once you learn to befriend yourself during all the different phases of progress that you go through, you will truly become unstoppable, and you'll find your flow in a much happier and healthier way.

And then you can *really* start to get stuff done.

Conclusion

As you've travelled through this book, hopefully you've learned to adopt a gentler approach to productivity, one that allows you enough space to rest, relax, focus, and play on a regular basis. We can learn to see all of these things as important to our general wellbeing, and we can make them our goals, too! We can learn to see taking care of ourselves each day as an essential part of how we get things done.

Most of all, I hope that by the end of this book, you've learned how to show yourself much more daily kindness, no matter what road you choose to travel down next.

Sometimes, we have to stop being so very busy to find our balance. And once we find that balance, we can tap into our amazing inner strength again.

Keep mapping out those goals and tell your brain exactly where you want to go next. Treat yourself with compassion every step of the way. Rest when you need to rest. Play when you need a break. Create enough space and time to focus when you need to get things done. Let yourself find your own unique flow that makes you feel happy and healthy as you start to do all the things that really matter to you.

I wish you all the best on your self-kindness journey ahead!

For more books by Risa Williams, including journals, audiobooks, and resources like worksheets related to the tools discussed in this book, please visit:
https://www.risawilliams.com/books.html

Follow Risa on Instagram: @risawilliamstherapy

Check out Risa's award-winning time management podcast, The Motivation Mindset:
https://podcasts.apple.com/us/podcast/the-motivation-mindset-with-risa-williams/id1643053152

If you'd like to work with Risa in time management coaching sessions, you can visit:
https://www.risawilliams.com/sessions.html

To join Risa's Get Stuff Done: Goals Group community, sign up at https://www.patreon.com/risawilliams

For monthly time management tips, videos, and free book giveaways, subscribe to Risa's newsletter at:
https://risa-williams.mailchimpsites.com/

Risa enjoys hearing from readers, so feel free to reach out to her by sending an email through her website at:
https://www.risawilliams.com/about.html.

She would love to hear what tips and tools from this book worked for you!

Acknowledgments

I'd like to thank all the wonderful readers of my books (including everyone reading this now), my clients and students, and my podcast audience for all of your kindness and support. Thank you to my wonderful kids, my loving husband, and my two cats for helping me find the fun while writing this book over the last year. Thanks to my amazing editor, Brenda Knight, for excitedly announcing, "Let's help the people bring their stress down!" when I first pitched this book to her, and for all of her work on this book, along with the production team at Mango, copy editor Artemisia L. Noble, and cover designer, Jodie Anders. Thanks to Jane Evans, Sean Townsend, and JKP Books, who published my previous books, *The Ultimate Toolkit Book Series* and *The Procrastination Playbook*. And a big thanks to friends and colleagues: Eden Byrne, Erica Curtis, Stevon Lewis, Sepideh Saremi, Dr. Scott Waltman, Mike Sonksen, Maggie Lynch, Andrew Lawston, Trevor Stockwell, Tšhegofatšo Ndabane, Miguel Chavez, Ryan Muldoon, Ezra Werb, Dr. Tamara Soles, Ramona Ortega, Christopher Cortman, Eric Maisel, Deanna Yates, Romy, Anton, and Veronica Yanagisawa, Joel Levin, Maja Starcevic, Dr. Catherine Smith, Kathryn Singer and Tony Smith, Hilary Kern, Jennifer Whitney, Holly Daniels, Chiwan Choi, Jay Fernandez, Alexis Hope, Gabby Sanderson, Dulcie Yamanaka, Michelle Jones, Amanda Way, and Deloss Brown.

I appreciate the kindness that all of you put out into the world, and I hope this book sends some kindness back to you, too. *For more books by Risa Williams, please visit www.risawilliams.com or follow her on Instagram @risawilliamstherapy. She enjoys hearing* from readers, so feel free to reach out to her through her website or leave an Amazon review.

For worksheets related to tools in this book, please visit: risawilliams.com.

References

Abramson, Ashley (2022) "Burnout and stress are everywhere." American Psychological Association, Vol. 53, No. 1, page 72.

Akimbekov, N.S. and Razzaque, M.S. (2021) "Laughter therapy: A humor-induced hormonal intervention to reduce stress and anxiety." *Current Research in Physiology 4*, 135-138. doi:10.1016/j.crphys.2021.04.002.

Bower, T. (2022) "Burnout is a Worldwide Problem: 5 Ways Work Must Change." *Forbes Magazine*, July 24, 2022. www.forbes.com/sites/tracybrower/2022/07/24/burnout-is-a-worldwide-problem-5-ways-work-must-change.

Can, Y.S., Iles-Smith, H., Chalabianloo, N., Ekiz, D., *et al.* (2020) "How to relax in stressful situations: A smart stress reduction system." *Healthcare 8*, 2, 100. doi:10.3390/healthcare8020100.

Chancellor, Gordon (editor), et al. *Charles Darwin's notebooks from the voyage of the Beagle.* Cambridge: University Press, 2009. (p. 598).

Chen, Ly (2024), "Writing things down may help you remember information more than typing." *New Scientist*, January 26th, 2024: www.newscientist.com/article/2414241-writing-things-down-may-help-you-remember-information-more-than-typing/.

Cherry, K. (2019) "How listening to music can have psychological benefits." *Very Well Mind*, December 10, 2019. www.verywellmind.com/surprising-psychological-benefits-of-music-4126866.

Contreras, C. M., and Gutiérrez-Garcia, A. G. (2018) "Cortisol awakening response: An ancient adaptive feature." *Journal of Psychiatry and Psychiatric Disorders 2*, 29-40. www.fortunejournals.com/articles/cortisol-awakening-response-an-ancient-adaptive-feature.html.

Goodin, R. E., Rice, J. M., Bittman, M., and Saunders, P. (2004) "The time pressure illusion: Discretionary time vs. free time." *Social Indicators Research 73*, 43-70. jamesmahmudrice.info/Time-Pressure.pdf.

Harvard University: Nutrition Source, *Stress and Health*, (2021) https://nutritionsource.hsph.harvard.edu/stress-andhealth/

Katzir, M., Emanuel, A., and Liberman, N. (2020) "Cognitive performance is enhanced if one knows when the task will end." *Cognition* 197, April, 2020, 104189. doi:10.1016/j.cognition.2020.104189.

Kok, B.E., Coffey, K.A., Cohn, M.A., Catalino, L.I., et al. (2013) "How positive emotions build physical health: Perceived positive social connections account for the upward spiral between positive emotions and vagal tone." *Psychological Science 24*, 7, 1123-1132. doi:10.1177/0956797612470827.

LaMotte, Sandee (2022) "Burnout may be changing your brain. Here's what to do." CNN Health, www.cnn.com/2022/03/10/health/burnout-changing-brain-wellness/index.html.

Fiorioni, S. and Foy, D. (2024) "Americans Sleeping Less, More Stressed." Gallup.com., April 15th, 2024. news.gallup.com/poll/642704/americans-sleeping-less-stressed.aspx.

Herz, Rachel (2016) "The Role of Odor-Evoked Memory in Psychological and Physiological Health," *Brain Sciences*, www.ncbi.nlm.nih.gov/pmc/articles/PMC5039451/pdf/brainsci-06-00022.pdf.

Jabr, F. (2013) "Why your brain needs more downtime." *Scientific American*, October 15, 2013. www.scientificamerican.com/article/mental-downtime.

Jaworksi, M. (2020) "The Negativity Bias: Why Bad Stuff Sticks." Health Central, Feb. 19, 2020. www.healthcentral.com/mental-health/negativity-bias.

Rothbard, N. P. and Wilk, S. L. (2011) "Waking up on the right or wrong side of the bed: Start-of-workday mood, work events, employee affect, and performance." *Academy of*

Management Journal, April 4, 2011. www.sciencedaily.com/releases/2011/04/110404151353. htm.

Ross, S. (2020) "How does stress affect your body?" *The American Institute of Stress*, February 10, 2020. www.stress.org/how-does-stress-affect-your-body-the-latest-research-shows-it-can-vary.

Ma, Xiao et al. (2017) "The Effects of Diaphragmatic Breathing on Attention, Negative Affect and Stress in Healthy Adults," *Frontiers in Psychology, Volume 8—2017*, www.frontiersin.org/journals/psychology/articles/10.3389/fpsyg.2017.00874/full.

Rothbard, N. P. and Wilk, S. L. (2011) "Waking up on the right or wrong side of the bed: Start-of-workday mood, work events, employee affect, and performance." *Academy of Management Journal*, April 4, 2011. www.sciencedaily.com/releases/2011/04/110404151353. htm.

Raghunathan, R. (2013) "How negative is your mental chatter?" *Psychology Today*, October 10, 2013. www.psychologytoday.com/us/blog/sapient-nature/201310/how-negative-is-your-mental-chatter.

Smith, Morgan (2023) "Harvard-Trained psychologist shares 3 Signs you're addicted to stress: It's a lot more common than you think." CNBC.com, www.cnbc.com/2023/05/07/harvard-trained-psychologist-reveals-3-signs-youre-addicted-to-stress.html.

University of the West of England (2018) "Coloring reduces stress and boosts creativity." Neuroscience News, May 4, 2018. neurosciencenews.com/coloring-stress-creativity-8969.

Vaughan, M. (2014) "Know your limits, your brain can only take so much." *Entrepreneur Magazine*. https://www.entrepreneur.com/living/know-your-limits-your-brain-can-only-take-so-much/230925.

White, M.P., Elliott, L.R., Grellier, J., and Economou, T. (2021) "Associations between green/blue spaces and mental health across 18 countries." *Scientific Reports 11*, 1, 8903. doi:10.1038/ s41598-021-87675-0.

Neuroscience News, Stanford University (2021) "Why multitasking does more harm than good," neuroscience.stanford.edu/ news/why-multitasking-does-more-harm-good.

Mental Health Resources

Psychotherapist Directories in the USA

Psychology Today: psychologytoday.com

Therapy Den: therapyden.com

Mental Health Organizations

Anxiety & Depression Association of America (ADAA): adaa.org

National Alliance on Mental Illness (NAMI) mental health hotlines (US): www.nami.org/Support-Education/NAMI-HelpLine/ Top-HelpLine-Resources

Mental Health Charities

National Alliance on Mental Illness: www.nami.org

Attention Deficit Disorder Organization: add.org

Brain & Behavior Research Foundation: www.bbrfoundation.org

Stress Reduction Strategies

Box breathing: psychcentral.com/health/box-breathing

American Institute of Stress: www.stress.org

Mindfulness

www.mindful.org

Grounding Techniques

www.choosingtherapy.com/grounding-techniques

Somatic Techniques for Stress Reduction

www.wellandgood.com/somatic-release-exercise

EMDR Butterfly Hug Technique

irp.cdn-website.com/4193fbeb/files/uploaded/soothing-butterfly-hug.pdf

Guided Meditation

www.mindful.org/how-to-meditate

Attention Deficit Disorder (ADD & ADHD) Tools

ADDitude Magazine: www.additudemag.com/category/adhd-add

Children and Adults with Attention Deficit (CHADD): chadd.org

howtoadhd.com

ADHD Self-Test: add.org/adhd-test

ADHD podcast and videos: drhallowell.com

Anxiety and Mental Health Resources

Anxiety & Depression Association of America (ADAA): adaa.org

Anxiety UK: www.anxietyuk.org.uk

Mind helpline: www.mind.org.uk/information-support/helplines

National Alliance on Mental Illness (NAMI) mental health hotlines (US): www.nami.org/Support-Education/NAMI-HelpLine/Top-HelpLine-Resources

Mindfulness Apps

Headspace: www.headspace.com

Calm: www.calm.com

Breathwork Apps

Othership: www.othership.us

One Deep Breath: https://odb.emercent.com

Focus-Based Online Groups

Focused Space: focused.space

Focusmate: focusmate.com

Get Stuff Done Goals Groups & Time Management Coaching Online

Risa Williams: risawilliams.com

EMDR (Eye Movement Desensitization and Reprogramming) & Somatic Therapy

EMDR Research Foundation: emdrresearchfoundation.org

General information on Somatic Therapy: www.health.com/somatic-therapy-7643892

Further Reading

The Procrastination Playbook for Adults with ADHD: How to Catch Sneaky Forms of Procrastination Before They Catch You by Risa Williams (Jessica Kingsley Books, 2024)

The Ultimate Time Management Toolkit: 25 Productivity Tools for Adults with ADHD and Chronically Busy People by Risa Williams (Jessica Kingsley Books, 2022)

The Ultimate Anxiety Toolkit: 25 Tools to Worry Less, Relax More, and Boost Your Self-Esteem by Risa Williams (Jessica Kingsley Book, 2021)

The Ultimate Self-Esteem Toolkit: 25 Tools to Boost Confidence, Achieve Goals, and Find Happiness by Risa Williams (Jessica Kingsley Books, 2023)

ADHD 2.0: New Science and Essential Strategies for Thriving with Distraction—from Childhood through Adulthood by Dr. Ned Hallowell and Dr. John J. Ratey (Ballantine Books, 2021)

Feeling Good: The New Mood Therapy by David D. Burns (William Morrow, 1999)

The Body Keeps the Score: Brain, Mind, and Body in the Healing of Trauma by Dr. Bessel van der Kolk (Penguin Books, 2020)

Atomic Habits: An Easy and Proven Way to Build Good Habits and Break Bad Ones by James Clear (Random House, 2018)

How to Relax (Mindfulness Essentials) by Thich Nhat Hanh (Parallax Press, 2015)

When the Body Says No: The Cost of Hidden Stress by Dr. Gabor Mate (Vermillion, 2019)

About the Author

Risa Williams is a licensed psychotherapist specializing in time management and goal-setting tools, a speaker, a psychology professor, a writer, and the award-winning author of five self-help books, including *The Ultimate Time Management Toolkit*, *The Ultimate Self-Esteem Toolkit*, *The Ultimate Anxiety Toolkit*, and *The Procrastination Playbook for Adults with ADHD*.

She's been interviewed and featured in many worldwide publications including *Forbes Magazine*, *Women's World*, *Wired Magazine*, *Business Insider*, *Very Well Mind*, *Psych Central*, *Therapist Magazine*, *L.A. Parent*, *Breathe Magazine*, *HuffPost*, and *Real Simple*. Her books have won three national awards, including the *Living Now Book Award*, and her podcast, *The Motivation Mindset*, received the *Positive Change Podcast Award*. She also runs Get Stuff Done Groups and trainings online. She lives with her husband and two kids in Los Angeles.

To read more by Risa, please visit risawilliams.com and follow her on Instagram @risawilliamstherapy. She enjoys hearing from readers—feel free to reach out to her through her website or Instagram.

A portion of the author's profits will be donated to National Alliance on Mental Illness (NAMI), a charity supporting mental health needs.

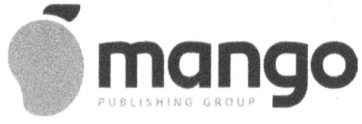

Mango Publishing, established in 2014, publishes an eclectic list of books by diverse authors—both new and established voices—on topics ranging from business, personal growth, women's empowerment, LGBTQ studies, health, and spirituality to history, popular culture, time management, decluttering, lifestyle, mental wellness, aging, and sustainable living. We were named 2019 *and* 2020's #1 fastest growing independent publisher by *Publishers Weekly*. Our success is driven by our main goal, which is to publish high-quality books that will entertain readers as well as make a positive difference in their lives.

Our readers are our most important resource; we value your input, suggestions, and ideas. We'd love to hear from you—after all, we are publishing books for you!

Please stay in touch with us and follow us at:

Facebook: Mango Publishing
Twitter: @MangoPublishing
Instagram: @MangoPublishing
LinkedIn: Mango Publishing
Pinterest: Mango Publishing
Newsletter: mangopublishinggroup.com/newsletter

Join us on Mango's journey to reinvent publishing, one book at a time.